ALSO BY THOMAS DEBAGGIO

Losing My Mind:
An Intimate Look at Life with Alzheimer's

WHEN IT GETS DARK

An Enlightened Reflection
on Life
with Alzheimer's

THOMAS DEBAGGIO

FREE PRESS
New York   London   Toronto   Sydney   Singapore

FREE PRESS
A Division of Simon & Schuster, Inc.
1230 Avenue of the Americas
New York, NY 10020

FREE PRESS and colophon are trademarks
of Simon & Schuster, Inc.

Designed by Jan Pisciotta

Manufactured in the United States of America

10 9 8 7 6 5 4 3 2 1

Library of Congress Cataloging-in-Publication Data

DeBaggio, Thomas
    When it gets dark : an enlightened reflection on life with Alzheimer's /
    Thomas DeBaggio.
    p. cm
    1. DeBaggio, Thomas, 1942—Mental health. 2. Alzheimer's disease—
        Patients—Virginia—Biography. I. Title
    RC523.D433 2003
    362.1'96831'0092—dc21
    [B]   2003049228

    ISBN 1-4165-7320-8

For information about special discounts for bulk purchases,
please contact Simon & Schuster Special Sales at
1-800-456-6798 or business@simonandschuster.com

To Joyce, my Muse, who encouraged me to follow my dream and then helped me to live this book, and to Francesco for whom I hope there is special meaning in these pages, and a long life. And especially to Ralph Morris who taught me the necessary things about humanity.

Acknowledgments

Joyce DeBaggio, my wife, and Francesco DeBaggio, my son, actively helped in writing this book. They were often my memory and they were always ready to walk with me as I struggled for words and memories that were now just beyond my horizon. It is no easy task to watch someone you love slowly revert to childlike behavior and worse. No one who has not faced Alzheimer's personally can know the secrets of the disease and its emotional pain and often bewilderment. Caregivers have the closest view of this mysterious, sorrowful, unwanted gift, and they are often the least acknowledged.

It was my good fortune several years ago to cross paths with Linda Ligon, as fine a friend and word maven as I have met. She surprised me one day with a gift, praise for my scribbles and a chance to share them with others. Later, she pushed me to poke in simple but dirty places, where I found overlooked meaning.

WHEN IT GETS DARK

Much of what we believe is mythical, a way to blur reality to make it easier to understand the past and how it connects with the present. We live on memories, whether it is a memory of how to replace a lightbulb or drive a car, or the recollection of our parents, lovers and children. The sum of our memories guide, befriend or leave us shivering with fear.

Memories, no matter how trivial, remind us of events and sorrows. They become a touchstone of who we were and who we want to be. The best we can do is rely on memory, acknowledging that not all of it is remembered well and faithfully.

You and I, we're both running against death, even when we can't touch it, or see its ugly face.

Cars swish beside me as I walk. The nervous titter of angry horns on speeding cars rushes by me. Pigeons gather on a single apartment roof at the same time each day awaiting my passage along the street.

THE APARTMENT WAS silent until the telephone splintered my solitude. I went to the kitchen and picked up the receiver.

Do you know where your wife is? an unfamiliar voice began.

Yes, I said. Who is this?

Right about now, the voice continued, she is in the arms of a big, nigger football player at the University of Delaware and she is panting as he sticks his big, black cock into her.

I hung up, exploding with fear and anger.

The telephone call was the first in a series I received. They often came when Joyce attended night meetings of the Wilmington Bail Committee, a community group established to help young black activists get out of jail on bond. It was the first time such a call truly frightened me.

I did not believe the words of the man on the telephone. What frightened me was someone in the dark watching, trying to disrupt our lives, maybe even tap our telephone. We were sure the phone calls came either from members of the Wilmington Police Department, members of the Delaware National Guard, or a special unit of the U.S. government on assignment after the city exploded with pent-up rage the day of Martin Luther King's assassination. Those who inhabited Wilmington during that time told stories of dark fear and trembling rage.

What brought me from the Midwest back to the East Coast and Wilmington was a job with a local daily newspaper, the

News Journal. It was here that my journalism dreams died. I stayed long enough at the newspaper to share a reporting award. We should have left town after those first six months at the newspaper, but the friends we made held us, at least for a while, and long enough for Francesco to complete first grade.

In Wilmington I encountered existential emptiness and for the first time I questioned the belief that America was the land of the free. For some, especially for African-Americans, it was an awkward, fearful hell if you dared challenge the status quo. When you are young, as we were then, you can see these things with frightful clarity.

Wilmington was an angry, segregated place, with African-Americans and whites living in separate and very unequal conditions. Fortunately, there were still those who believed in the promise freedom held for all. I remember a woman living outside Wilmington, who left her front door unlocked to give those on the run a place to eat and sleep, the way African-Americans fled the slave masters of years ago. From what she told me, it seemed the old underground railroad was alive and well, with a crowded stop at her home. There were few others with the same reckless spirit.

These were tough, outrageous times and it brought out the best of some people in Wilmington. It was a rare chance to rip back layers of fear and watch dedicated individuals work to release those in quiet bondage. Also during this time, I watched with tearful eyes what could have been the best and brightest of Wilmington succumb to the deadly evils of heroin, surely one of the "dirtiest" ways to silently disarm an angry young population of black men and women.

Tears tumble uncontrolled across my cheeks as I sit in the living room chair. What calls the tears to lubricate my cheeks? Where is the secret pain that causes this outpouring of sorrow?

*   *   *

Joyce and I, and a bewildered six-year-old Francesco, gathered our belongings and ran from the fears of Delaware like peasants fleeing a plague. We left behind some of the best friends we ever had, but we could not handle the political pressures and the frightening calls in the middle of the night. It was a place in which strong currents pushed us to be people we were not. We were not skilled in this kind of combat.

We returned to Virginia, the one place we knew best, with tears in our eyes. It was home for both of us, the place where Joyce and I grew up in our own separate and peculiar ways. Even if we weren't at home, it was a place we understood. Here we licked our wounds and bemoaned the loss of so many good friends left behind. The spirit of our friends in Delaware was not far away and we could make short forays across the border to be with them.

We shacked up in a dreary huddle of brick, two-story attached houses on the underskirts of well-off Alexandria, Virginia. Our back side was against a large shopping center. Through our back window and the broken wooden fence, we saw men and women heft themselves into a green dumpster in search of their daily sustenance. They sifted carefully through the out-of-date food the Giant grocery tossed away every day. The smell from the container was sometimes rich with rotting food, and bees and flies worked their way through the soft, rotting remains.

THERE ARE DAYS full of static when little memory remains, and I wander over the hidden landscape like a child trying to catch slippery raindrops. The interior cacophony I carry within me is full of broken sentences, and tears.

There are other days when memory is so thick and beautiful I can't see the world for all the happy congestion.

So this is the way my world ends, fighting shadows, wrapped in fear, trembling to remember who I am and where I am headed.

Despite the poverty of words, and a memory chewed by Alzheimer's, I intend to open my inner life and at the same time reflect on everyday simple things, as death's shadow falls across my dwindling days. This is not a book of kings and queens but of ordinary people struggling in the world they inhabit. It is my world, and the world of my wife, Joyce, and son, Francesco.

This is not a book crafted with care and threaded with hope. It is a book of anger and tears, expressed in a cage of waiting death ruled by Alzheimer's, a disease without survivors.

I became a creature of the tension between a life of the moment and the languid, rotting fruit of memory upon which I rely for life.

This is not a book barren of trees, birds and ordinary sweat.

In the end, this book is about becoming silent, while all around cars honk impatiently.

❧

Our move from Delaware was made possible by Ted Rowse, a publisher of consumer affairs newsletters in Washington, D.C. I met him at a convergence of muckrakers and we shared stories. I was unaware he was sizing me up for a job on a newsletter to be called *Consumer Newsweek.*

When Ted's call came offering me a job, we lacked the money to move and he paid our expenses. I went to work right away in a little two-room office in the National Press Building in the heart of Washington, D.C., two blocks from the White House. Consumer consciousness was raised daily during the early 1970s by Ralph Nader. He was the shining light of the time, building a muckraking empire to right wrongs. There was an aura of hope, and change was in the air.

From the first day on Rowse's payroll, life became wondrous. What a job it was for a young journalist. It required covering Congress and dashing around town in cabs to attend press conferences held in gray government offices.

Rowse's office was on the seventh floor and I looked down on the street and saw throbbing movement everywhere. Computers were not even in our dreams and big manual typewriters were what we used to produce the newsletters. It was the first job in which I felt secure and happy.

It never occurred to me we had to find subscribers to support my journalism. It was a lesson I learned quickly. The grant money Ted used to hire me ran out long before the newsletter found a following. I loved the job so much I worked for nothing for several months after Ted told me he could no longer pay me.

I was able to stay on for a few more months because Joyce found a job with a shop-at-home company making custom slipcovers and window treatments. She went out to homes and helped the owners choose the coverings and fabrics. She was able to set her own schedule and worked around Francesco's school hours.

I hoped for a miracle but it didn't come. After a short 10-month stay, I was suddenly a flash in the pan and out of journalism again.

At night my days are stolen, leaving me weeping for even a glimmer of yesterday.

Now, NEARLY THIRTY years after we fled Wilmington, my body, burdened by time, has begun to disintegrate in subtle and angry ways, as my brain slowly turns into Alzheimer's mush. I find myself in yet another battle, this time from a combatant I cannot see.

Like old window glass, buffeted by slashing rain, blurred images fill the sorrowful world of my days. At night, when I shut my eyes to sleep, I am sometimes bombarded with hallucinations. They appear first as flashing lights of many colors, sometimes greens, and blues predominate. A few moments later white klieg lights spin brightly to the surprise of my shut eyes. In these uncontrollable moments, hallucinations overtake my brain. If it were real, my eyes would burn from the heat. In these private moments I see things all around me, unseen by everybody else. Sometimes the hallucinations are so weak they turn into still photographs in which individuals, stiff from invincible time, pose for the camera as in times past.

It is hard to make sense of the world under these conditions. If I viewed the world through blurred images of old window glass, I might believe I inhabit a universe of fearful, angry currents.

My world today has all the strangeness of the flowing images of an underwater world. Sometimes I try to read a sentence but several of the words appear unfamiliar. If I stare at the word long enough, I am usually able to understand its meaning.

Six months ago my reading comprehension was quite ordinary. That was before my vocabulary began to totter and slip into the oil tank of perdition. Many more waves of destruction are yet to come, ending in a humiliating ball of frightful, child-like confusion.

Small insults occur every day, most of them centered on loss of vocabulary, but I have trouble understanding television as well. I am creeping on two legs toward a world of crawling and diapers.

* * *

A robin dances lightly along the overhead power line. With a nimble bounce it dives into the dense, green-leaved bay tree covering the side of the house where a nest hides.

❧

W<small>HEN WE RETURNED</small> to Virginia, the place we called home, we put Francesco in public school. He did well in first grade in Delaware but before long we discovered he was doing poorly. Francesco said he didn't understand what was going on. I fired off a letter to his second grade teacher. He came from an open classroom situation and the teacher thought Francesco understood how things worked. Unfortunately, the two open classrooms were different. Once he understood the new system, his grades improved.

Before long Christmas brought new hurdles. We told Francesco early in his life Santa Claus was make-believe but now he was confused; his teacher talked about Santa Claus as if he were real. I sent a second letter to his teacher, urging her to tell the truth about Santa.

Later, Joyce and I talked with the teacher but she offered no solution. Life was against our desire to be truth tellers. Francesco's teacher must have thought me a madman-dreamer, an out-of-control Don Quixote. She was probably right.

As Francesco grew older, his fascination with Christmas trees sharpened. I tried to divert him by decorating dead tree branches one year. Finally I gave in and bought an artificial tree on sale. It didn't assuage Francesco's need for a real tree that dropped needles and made a mess.

I was never able to weaken Francesco's love of Christmas. He celebrates now with the biggest tree his house will hold, but he doesn't stay up late on Christmas Eve waiting for Santa.

Joyce and I still have the plastic tree but it stays in the basement
unused.

An epiphany of wonder brings a raw, grisly, blunt
shout from my anxious throat, the loud, rough honking
of Alzheimer's, revealing a sudden hidden emotion com-
pounded by fear, and weakening mortality.

After I quit writing consumer journalism, I wrote pieces again
for the *Delaware Spectator.* I helped Ralph Morris start the paper
when we lived in Wilmington and I kept in touch with him by
phone and on occasional visits. I took the train to and from
Wilmington. Tuesdays I took a seven A.M. train from Union Station in Washington to Wilmington. I returned Thursday night.

I bunked next door to Ralph in his brother's house on West
10th Street. I never saw much of brother Joe, a schoolteacher,
but the front door was always unlocked and I was glad to have
the use of his spare bedroom. Dorina, Ralph's wife, always had
supper waiting for us but she never knew when we'd show up at
night.

Ralph tried to pay me regularly but the paper was not making money. I received several checks for $100, but the newspaper
was draining Ralph financially and physically. When Ralph
paid me he always reminded me how shaky the newspaper's
financial footing was. Be sure to cash the check before you leave
Wilmington, he always cautioned.

I loved working with Ralph and Trader and Van Riper, and
the characters who dropped in the newspaper's little office. It
broke my heart when I told Ralph I had accepted a job as night
editor at the *Northern Virginia Sun,* the Arlington newspaper on
which I cut my journalistic teeth in high school.

I talk in hollow rooms, awake to brain and sinew, but
I get lost easily in my mind and forget the words before

they are spoken. It is the first whisper of a shattering experience to come. It is called Alzheimer's but it is slow strangulation in a silence of its own.

❋

SLEEP NO LONGER comes easily. I awake in the night often now, as never before. In the bedroom at night the air is thick with tiny dark specks vibrating in the air, although Joyce says she cannot see them. Occasionally, this dark thick air is pierced by the waving of tattered yellow flags that flash on and off as they slide around the ceiling and along the upper reaches of the walls. It sometimes seems I am witnessing the ritual burning of yesterday's dreams and events. Joyce says she has never seen the midnight light show and I presume I am hallucinating.

Until three weeks ago, nights were not full of sleeplessness and fear. Now almost every night is full of screams and distress. Unless I note it on the pad of paper next to the bed, I have no memory of it in the morning.

In a strange way, the visual movement of the air and the steady sound of the window air conditioner are becoming as calming as an old friend. I view the increasing hallucinations and difficulty sleeping as new markers on my way into the forever-dark of Alzheimer's.

Another robin prepares a grassy nest under the inside eave of the greenhouse. She hops around the nest in anticipation, putting everything in order. A long skein of dried grass dangles from the little nest.

My cat Sabina is in the kitchen, perched inside the open window behind the kitchen sink, while I prepare breakfast. I turn at the high-pitched stuttering sound she emits. She is alerting me to the presence of a bird. The bird balances carefully on a skinny dark branch of a big ornamental tree reaching almost to the eves.

The thickly branched trees along the side of the house are often hiding places for birds and druids. As I approach the window, the bird nervously takes off and buries itself in the dense foliage along the tall fence hiding us from the used car lot. Sabina, barred by the screen, tenses and is ready to take off after the bird. She begins making small noises out of frustration when she realizes it has gotten away again.

Three little greenish-blue eggs lie in a nest snugged high in the greenhouse on a piece of gray conduit. Mama robin's feathery body warms them.

I WAS STILL thinking traditionally, and I saw the job at the *Sun* as the start I needed to send me back into daily journalism and a good job at a large paper. Joyce was making money with her shop-at-home job, although there were aspects of it she disliked, and we had just received money from the lawyer in Iowa who was handling my mother's estate. The amount was not large, especially when split with my sister, but now we had money, and we were both settled in jobs. We started looking for a house to buy.

Joyce did the legwork with a realtor. Together they looked at many places but could not find the perfect house. Joyce scoured the classified ads and one day she took me to see a house on North Ivy Street in Arlington. The house was empty and locked, but we liked what we saw from the porch through the big bay window, especially the fireplace and the big room around it.

The real estate agent later took us inside the house. We noticed how the shiny old wood flooring slanted in the upstairs bedrooms. The house was owned by an old woman who lived out of town and paid an agent to care for her many real estate investments. In the negotiations that ensued, Joyce managed to bring the price down, and we bought it with a down payment that came from my mother's estate. Payments were low, under a hundred dollars a month, but a large balloon payment required full payment in ten years.

Three eggs have hatched. The robin sits on the edge of the nest and presents a long red worm to the new arrivals.

INSTEAD OF DIFFICULT work with words in the stillness of my writing room, I secretly find my way to the Mossy Creek of my imagination, a little, meandering stream in Virginia, and cast to the rising trout of my dreams. These pleasant moments of vicarious fishing take me to a world of make-believe where the slow-moving creek is full of eager, big fish. A long rod and a tiny fly bring relaxation and quiet contemplation. In the late afternoon, I stare at the computer screen and watch a make-believe sun fulfill my secret dreams.

The robin slips in and out of the greenhouse through the open roof vents. She is watchful, slow and determined. Three mouths chirp for food.

JOYCE AND I moved our meager belongings from the apartment in Bradlee to the house on Ivy Street. Everything we owned didn't come close to filling the rental truck.

It was a mild day for December, and the friends who helped

us move were gone by early afternoon. After they left, Joyce and I sat in the nearly bare living room, proud of ourselves and full of dreams. This shaded, old structure now incubated our dreams, while our young son, Francesco, grew into a man.

In our reverie, we could not overwhelm the cold December air slowly insinuating itself into the living room. It was not long before we noticed our jackets were impotent to warm us. We threw a log or two into the little fireplace with the white wooden surround. Almost immediately the room filled with smoke. It was then we realized the fireplace, intended to draw warm smoke through its chimney, was unworkable. In time we learned the first tenant of the house had left quickly because of the house's persistent cold.

The heating system, installed in the mid-1920s, was not working and we made a call to an unknown heating specialist. He was at our house quickly, went into the basement, and assessed the situation. A small part had failed and he went through the alley across the street and came back with the necessary part. The old gas furnace still provides us with warmth.

The house, built before 1920, was the worse for wear, in spite of the work done to prepare the house for sale. The sagging wallpaper covering the ceilings was thickened with white stippling, making the ceiling look like an upside down sandbox. We pretended the fresh paint with which the previous owner anointed the walls and ceilings made the old house new.

When you don't ask questions, the world empties.

Many past occupants of our house left signs of their residence. None was more intriguing than what we uncovered in the basement. It became a place to search for artifacts of yesteryear. We looked at the basement, for all its rough-and-ready feel, the way Columbus may have seen the New World.

In a dark angle next to a brick chimney sat a huge furnace

with a web of thick pipes sprouting in all directions. It was here we made our first contact with something like history. The furnace was made by a company bankrupted in the early 1930s, according to the repairman who visited us when it failed to work.

Here we were in the mid-1970s sorting through the history of a little-remembered house built somewhere around 1918 and we find another hidden harvest. Some of the heavy paper wrapped around the heating pipes for warmth was beginning to decay, revealing rolls of newspaper underneath. Clearly someone who lived in this house tried to make the heating system more efficient.

The same heating system still warms our radiators, and the many pipes emanating from it appear to be something of a crumbling archive. Today the archive that wraps the heating pipes is as unread as it was when we moved in the house.

This morning I went to the basement wondering how long these newspapers might have been wrapped around the heating pipes. I carefully removed the heavy outer paper and found a rolled page from the December 22, 1938, *Washington Evening Star*. It contained an Associated Press report with a headline that read, "Crop Board Reports Lower Wheat Harvest."

Death comes in slow motion to many of us with Alzheimer's. Sometimes I wish the disease would hurry up and be done with. Waiting to die in confusion while your memory shivers away is like living out your last days in an uncomfortable refrigerator.

Prior to our residence in the house, it was let to a variety of eager, impecunious young people. In the basement, young men rented a concrete floor. They did little to hide the rough concrete block walls. A plastic curtain hung over an open drain for a shower. A hose from an inside spigot attached to a cement sink provided water. A tiny water closet wrapped in loose, rough boards held an old toilet and a sink with running water. Sheets hung for privacy from thick, bare rafters.

I am followed by images of death.

It must have been tough to live there when it rained. There were open holes in the concrete, and in a heavy rain, water and thick yellow dirt oozed up through the openings and spread all over the floor.

Upstairs a group of women shared another level of the house, occupying the three bedrooms and bath upstairs and a commodious kitchen, dining room and living room on the first floor. Fifteen locks carefully secured the basement door. The women took no chances on midnight visitations from the men living in the basement.

The robin makes many trips and is sometimes gone for long periods. One day while she is gone, I take a look in the nest. Two baby robins are dead. The third is gone. Death follows in my wake.

Moving day was exhausting and happy, but it was also frightening. After we returned the rental truck, we got in the car and drove out to Annandale, where Joyce's parents lived. We left many boxes, and piles of unglazed pottery, with them when we went to Delaware. Many of these wonders, pieces of my unfinished clay, remained in the Annandale garage for years, awaiting emancipation. Tag ends of my youthful enthusiasm with clay continue to float into our lives from time to time but its lively memory has slowly eroded over the years, turning dreams into unremembered quaintness.

While Joyce and I sorted the boxes and placed them in the car, Francesco, then about seven, was inside the house with his grandfather. Suddenly, an upset Francesco appeared.

Grandpa won't play with me, he said.

We hurried into the house. Joyce's father was having a heart attack. We got him into the car and drove him to the hospital. We made it in the nick of time. Although his heart had stopped, the doctors brought him back to life.

The heart attack brought light and reality into our young lives, as had my parents' deaths. The frightening fragility of living hovered above us at a time when invincibility appeared everywhere in our lives.

Joyce's father recovered, and there were several more heart attacks over the next twenty years until cruel time and tears caught up with him, strapped to a hospice bed.

Sometimes my brain speeds away on its own, prospecting for memories to hold me through the night. I see snapshots of people as they speed by on a circular road, nameless faces with unknown eyes. Can I tell if they are real from the fleeting impression I have of these hurried moments before I fall asleep?

My days are full of searching for what I no longer remember.

Acres of lush farmland and cherry orchards were sacrificed to build the houses in the old development in which we live. Many of the dwellings in this area were constructed before sewers ran under streets. Instead pipes routed the sewage to underground septic tanks, in our case to a place near the back of the property.

Horse-drawn carts with large metal tanks arrived solemnly to pump the underground waste and hauled it away. One of the waste hauling services could be seen from the room in which I sit. When horses died, they were buried on the property next to ours, now a block-long used-car lot. All the commercial space around us is filled with shiny, used automobiles and with companies repairing used cars.

The first people who lived in what is now our house were newlyweds but they did not stay long. The house was built for them but they were unhappy from the first day they occupied it, although the living room was outfitted with a large heating stove. The stovepipe was connected to an inadequate chimney, and the room often filled with smoke, as it did that day we first inhabited the house.

History also inhabited the area near where this old house stands. A short block from where Ivy Street dead-ends, Pershing Drive cuts a straight swath through the community of elderly homes, ending at the gates of Fort Myer, the precursor of the giant Pentagon, America's war room.

When the Wright brothers came to show America's military mandarins their new flying machine, it was over what is now Pershing Drive that they flew an early model of their famous plane.

The reservoir of memory soon disappears and even the sound of breathing becomes unfamiliar.

On our side of Ivy Street there is still no sidewalk for several blocks. We pretend it is part of the charm of the street. More important, the houses were sited too close to the street. If our roadway were widened, the sidewalk would come against our front steps, ending what little privacy we have.

Even where the street is wide enough, and sidewalks are present, hardly anybody walks on them. On both sides of the street, the denizens of our neighborhood hurry to work in the morning and return in the evening, sauntering down the middle of the dispirited asphalt. It has been this way for at least the thirty years we have lived here.

It has taken a while for me to understand the meaning of walking in the street instead of on sidewalks. I think it provides a way to intellectually maintain the idea that we live in small town America. This conceit is necessary now that we look into the sky and see a swinging horizon choked with twenty-story-high buildings, muscling their way into our skyline.

The street played an important role in the community in earlier times, too. An old-timer told me many years ago that the driver of a car going down Ivy Street on a weekend had to be careful not to maim someone because heads and feet were scattered all along the street under cars. The limbs belonged to the men who lived in the houses along Ivy Street and they entertained themselves on weekends greasing themselves under their cars parked along the street.

The neighborhood has changed markedly since then. The men no longer huddle under cars on their backs, awaiting weekend oily forgiveness. Now, in a bow to gasoline and the past, the newcomers push loud lawn mowers in endless circles. They kick up dirt and leaves in an attempt to manicure lawns with dreams of their own inner world, an outsized place of order and control.

What makes an eighty-year-old man keep a photograph of an overnight woman he knew fleetingly half a century ago in wartime Europe? Why does he insist on showing it to me with a wink while his wife sits with us?

One of the first things we discovered was the hobby of a man down Ivy Street from our house. He had a hankering for antique cars. The oldest vehicle in his garage was a spotless, black Model T. He spent many weekend hours working on it and his other cars. Eventually, he got the old antique working and on weekends he backed the Model T out of his long skinny driveway and toured the neighborhood with the top down. It was a way to air out all the years the car remembered, like walking a dog, only cleaner. The old car rattled a little and it did not have the smooth, muscular sound found purring under the hood of a late-model auto, but it had a head-turning quotient that was worth millions. The old car stays in the garage most of the time these days, awaiting show-off days to come.

When I die nothing will be left except someone else's memory of me. Only these words of mine will remain to shred my life into moments I now quickly forget.

I disliked the night shift at the *Northern Virginia Sun*. Most of the work was organizational. I oversaw the final production of the paper and did rewrite work for the next day's edition. It may not have been the job I coveted but I thought it was a move in the right direction. I still managed to send the *Spectator* a few articles but they were rarely Delaware based and lacked the hard-hitting quality for which I was known.

I thought things were going well at the *Sun* until the managing editor mentioned to me the publisher was unhappy that certain photographs and press releases were not appearing on the front page where he wanted them. I saw no news value to most of the press releases and they were not of front page importance.

The managing editor enlightened me with a note left on my desk one night. The photographs and press releases were of special importance to the publisher, I was informed, and they must be placed on page one. They highlighted the businesses or events of the publisher's friends. I paid the memo little attention. By that time I had quite a few of these press releases in the slush pile.

Several weeks passed and I continued to pay little attention to putting press releases on the front page. I was surprised one morning to see the publisher come in the front door just before I was to leave. He talked to me pointedly about his friends and why he wanted to promote their businesses. He was declaiming and picking his nose and working up a sweat over this.

I finally saw how important this was for him but I also realized how venal and unprofessional it was. I saw no reason a small local paper should not have the same professional values as larger organizations. Integrity is the cornerstone of all communication. I resigned on the spot and walked the three blocks home. It was several days before Christmas.

I am the protector of bad dreams.

❀

I sit in the silent darkness of the early morning and whisper to myself, sometimes of mortality and its faults. At other times, the early morning darkness makes me smile and I start to whistle but hold back; I do not want to awaken Joyce.

In these early morning moments I feel most alive. The only other times I feel like this is when the writing is going well and I look at the words as they blow out before me on the screen, as if my silent voice called them into being. These happy times are usually moments I delete because I want to own this time myself.

The water in the small stream slips by, cleaning the rocks with a happy burbling sound. I sense something familiar and happy deep inside me is gone.

I spent the summer traveling. I got halfway across my back yard.

—Louis Agassiz

❧

THERE WAS TIME the first year on Ivy Street, when I was out of work, to watch the shape of clouds in the sky. Day after day time stood still, allowing me to look down a glorious kaleidoscope through which to remember the rich, dark gold of the past and compare it to the empty, glittering pleasures of the present.

It was a time to be young, married and out of work, and maintain a feeling of carelessness without guilt. It was a time of sad inherited riches from parents too early dead amidst the disheartening turbulence of war in Vietnam.

It was a time of rupture on the home front as generations collided, smashing loving relationships over wartime disputes. Fear of war and dying propelled rifts that never healed. My parents died too young, before the war ended and permitted us to love each other again fully, or let them appreciate their baby grandson.

It was also a time when being recently orphaned, a catastrophe that happens to nearly all of us, no longer brought secret tears in the night. This was a time and a place when I thought it was possible to build a life around hope and a garden full of fresh vegetables.

My days are full of anxiety and searching, for what I no longer remember.

The house was new to our language and ignorant of our ways. It was going to take time to discipline this place and get used to living in a new world. We had some money, probably enough to get us through the winter. There was time to look for a job. In the meantime, there was work around the house.

From the front, the house was an old sweet wooden beauty, but hidden away in the backyard was sin city, a place where grass was cut infrequently and every calamity had been welcomed. If there were secrets to be uncovered, it was in this shambling, disordered backyard.

Little saplings, many grown large, weaved their tendrils through the rusting wire fencing that marked the boundary with our neighbors. The house on one side of us was owned by a naval officer who rented it to tenants who did little to keep it up. Opposite the renters, a tall wooden fence and towering trees provided a visual barrier from our business neighbors, who used a large square block to sell used cars. Directly behind us was a small white house with a mother, father and two boys about Francesco's age.

January was mild and clear that year and being out of work gave me the opportunity to begin to put our stamp on the place. A garage from a long ago era of short, narrow cars stumbled like a disreputable drunk in our backyard. Its last use had been to house a pair of large dogs; black bunches of hair were everywhere. From the alterations the animals undertook, it appeared they enjoyed the makeshift dwelling too much.

The front of the building hung wide open and the large single door was askew. Holes were smashed in the side of the structure, either by the dogs or their keepers, and it gave the place an angry, open feeling. Even the concrete pad was ruptured, with deep cracks rippling through it like deep wounds. Eyesore was the first description that came to mind.

The wood from which the garage was constructed was thin and the uprights to which it was attached were skinny. With a couple of hard shoves, the old garage collapsed into a dirty pile of wood and thick dust. An unhealthy stench rose in the air. Joyce's father helped me put the wooden pieces of the old garage on the sidewalk to be taken away. The concrete had to be broken with heavy sledgehammers, work I saved for later.

Saplings were growing everywhere along the fence line. Some as tall as ten feet were well established. These had to be cut in many places and dug from the ground. Many tree trunks swelled around the thick metal fencing. Cutting the tops of these saplings, and in some cases more mature trees, became a struggle between me and nature.

I spent days, weeks, months, sweating as the sun heated the earth. There were days spent untangling a single thick sapling and cutting it into pieces small enough to handle. Digging roots entangled in the fencing took the longest time.

The work was particularly difficult along the back of the property where our neighbor had a chain-link fence. There were moments I wished I had a bomb to blow the long metal pipes out of the earth.

For relaxation, I marked off a garden plot, stripped the sod, which was mostly weeds, and put it on the side of the house facing the car lot where a driveway had been before the county installed a new sidewalk, blocking what little remained of the driveway.

In a long, wide, sunny place in the backyard I staked an area to grow enough vegetables to see us through the year. I sowed a wide variety of seed, everything from beets and cabbage to tomatoes and corn and lots of quick little stuff, chard, radishes, and an assortment of lettuces. My attachment to herbs was in the future.

Neighborhood watch: A man pulled along by a huge dog passes my front window. Behind the man a woman marches along carefully holding a paper sack that appears to be full of dog droppings.

One day I looked up from smashing what remained of the garage concrete to find my neighbor leaning on her rusting wire fence. I smiled and walked to greet her.

I've been watching you work in the yard for several days, she said. What are you planning?

She was a short, solid woman with dark black hair. I saw her two lively boys playing in her backyard. They were about the same age as Francesco.

I'm turning this backyard into a garden, I said. There will be vegetables there. I pointed to the middle of the yard, stripped of grass and awaiting the next assignment. I didn't mention that the garden was needed to supply us with most of what we would eat that summer, fall and winter.

Over there I want a little pond, I said, pointing toward the back of her peeling, white garage that backed up to the property line.

Oh, she said. We always liked the trees.

I was startled that someone on the other side would complain about the rickety absence of the self-sown saplings in my yard. I had also torn out a crumbling pile of bricks, once an outdoor barbecue, I considered an eyesore. It turned out she liked that, too.

My new neighbor, having informed me I ruined the view from her back window, turned abruptly and walked back to her house. It never occurred to me it might be necessary, or even polite, to consult with my neighbors before I did a general cleanup. It was the first of many such lessons to come.

Alzheimer's is like a bad dream sneaking up behind me, filling my portals with death and destruction.

I had a huge and hurried appetite for a garden after being confined to rented apartments and townhouses for several years. Within six weeks of moving, the backyard was cleared of the ramshackle garage and broken concrete, and my dream of a garden began. Surely we had discovered Eden or some other paradise.

Maple saplings wove themselves through the wire fences and I cut them down before I stepped off the space for the garden. What was the hurry? The sun poured into this tender spot of fecund earth and gave it energy and warmth.

The first spring garden was begun by peeling back the green stuff called grass. It was rolled into fat brown earthen sausages. This sod was transplanted to a bare area on the north side of the house to cover the gravel driveway. When there was no longer a place to transplant sod, I dumped bags for the trash collector. I discovered later the top portion I was so eager to save was filled with large, succulent, wiry white roots of irreclaimable perennial Bermuda grass.

With an old dime store spade with a wobbly handle, I was determined to double-dig this huge area and add copious piles of humus to soften the hard clay and improve tilth and drainage. As I worked my way steadily across the back from north to south parallel to the fence, the spade came to a jolting stop about eighteen inches down. I had already unearthed buried treasure in the form of old bottles, buttons, boulders and French drains, but this time the shovel didn't budge. When I could not go around the obstacle easily, I tried to uncover it like an archeologist. There was an intentional structure under the spot where my garden was to be and I thought at first I had unearthed an old foundation of historical interest.

My romantic ideas of what lay under this corner of the garden were soon dashed when my neighbor, who was watching me with wonder, leaned across the fence and told me it was the site of an old septic system. There was no use trying to remove the remnant of the half-century-old sewage system. I mounded the earth around it and made use of the fertility deposited there.

I still remember the tomato plants marching along in measured formation, the broccoli planted so excitedly. In early March the cold wind shredded and blackened many leaves, the lettuces, the beets, the cabbages, the cauliflower, the squashes, the cucumbers and all the rest. But it is the old septic system that lies solidly under the earth that holds a monumental place in my memory. Discovering it has always held a special meaning for me because it is the only thing I have unearthed that is solid and has a trace of a story attached to it. There is something sweet in planting a garden over a rich archeological site.

There are few old-timers left who remember how things were in 1917 when the old cherry orchard became inhabited with houses, including ours. There is almost nobody who remembers where the old septic tanks were located and how the rudimentary sewage system worked, and before long it will be a memory no one has.

I wonder what future gardeners will think when their spades come to a sharp, jolting stop against underground concrete while preparing the soil in what is now my backyard. How puzzled this new gardener will be to find three-foot-deep columns of concrete 14 inches wide. What use could these have been? they may wonder. Will they ever discover the underground artifacts that hold my greenhouse and sheltered thousands of plants for hundreds of people who trekked here to buy them? There may be somebody around who remembers but the new occupants of my backyard will never know how much fun I had on this little bit of earth.

This earth lived long before us and it will live long after us and it tells many stories. Its tales are not always in an understandable language. As long as humans live on this planet, there will be plants, whether weeds or more intentional plantings. Those who know the meaning of what lies beneath the sod will draw sustenance from the rich mulch of the past.

I am bewildered every day in secret ways. Forces I never knew existed have taken over places in my body. Alzheimer's works silently but its evil is steady, drilling through my brain until I no longer trust myself.

While the garden grew, I put my efforts into temporary work. I bought a lawn mower and leafleted every house for several blocks, extolling my expertise at cutting grass, trimming shrubs and other hard work. I felt secure, and in my youth I was overconfident.

Not more than half a dozen neighbors were interested in my services. Some of the lawn mowing was only temporary during vacations. I waddled through the hot, sweaty summer cutting a few lawns, but it was clear I was not going to make a living cutting grass and doing handyman jobs.

It has not been long since I last looked into the chaos of the abyss and cried. Now that tarnished world beckons again. I loosen shards from the steep walls to begin my long descent into the lonely world of silence. It is a world so secret its vocabulary has not been written.

Francesco was not averse to work and he helped me dig and polish the landscape. He missed the Bradlee paper route and the money it provided. When an *Evening Star* route opened, Francesco was on the top of the list, thanks to his last route supervisor, who praised his work. The *Star* was an afternoon paper and Francesco hurried home from fifth grade to walk the two long streets of his territory.

I delivered papers as boy and man, and Francesco and I knew the pitfalls, the families who moved without paying, or worse, the people who wouldn't pay but insisted on newspaper delivery. He had some unusual, tough customers.

This was an era of manipulated sophistry when boys (and a few girls) were considered entrepreneurs by large, wealthy American newspaper companies. The newspaper hired drivers to deliver their newspapers to children who carried them to homes. The children collected the money due at the end of the month. If the customers down the street didn't pay, the child newspaper carriers paid for them and were often cheated.

It was frustrating enough for Francesco to spend night after night trying to find customers home and willing to pay. He came home complaining after many nights spent trying to collect the money owed him. People were away for the evening often; but worse were the customers who had no excuses for not paying and used Francesco's money as a no-interest loan.

He had two men who were so difficult we fired them. One of them was at the end of Ivy Street, a single man who was not there or didn't have any money to pay him. After six months of trying, I went with Francesco. He treated me the same way he treated my son. He owed for six months of Sunday papers. When he wouldn't pay, I told him Francesco wouldn't deliver.

A second customer lived in a basement reached through an alley across the street from us. He was well spoken and traveled a lot, but he too didn't have money to pay. Francesco stopped delivering his Sunday paper.

Bad pays were not the only hazards. There was one customer slightly off his route but easily reached, if you wanted to walk up several flights of stairs. The apartment was one of many in a two- or three-floor walk-up. Francesco had to deliver there only Sunday, but he never wanted to go in, knock on the door and collect what was due. I offered to accompany him one evening. Francesco was right, the place smelled like a chicken farm, or worse. He knocked and a woman opened the door. The stench was overpowering. In the background I saw dozens of cats walking around the room and on top of the fireplace.

One night Francesco came back near tears. He had parked his bike and gone up to the house. The people asked him in while they wrote a check for the month's newspapers. In those few moments inside, Francesco's bike was stolen in the dark.

Francesco had a hunch who might have stolen it but it wasn't for many years that the boy down the street, now a man, come back to visit his past. He confessed to me he took the bike.

I don't think many of his customers knew how dedicated Francesco was to delivering their newspapers. At least not until a winter snowstorm dumped 20 inches of snow over several days. There is a photo somewhere in the house of Francesco leaving home the day after the snowfall with his trusty newspaper bag loaded up, struggling through snow up to his waist.

White stones glistening in the sun. Mossy stones climbing up a steep hill. Boulders snug in soft moss. A blinding white light fades supernaturally as I shut my eyes to sleep.

❊

MY CAT SABINA is less like a feline and more like a human than any animal I have come across. In her deafness she has developed a special language of sound and pointing through which she talks to me. When she wants food, she goes to the kitchen and sits in front of the cabinet door where her food is stored. She rubs the side of the door with her head several times. If I don't respond, she lets out a supernatural scream that gets my attention immediately.

It is hard to shake the uneasiness I feel, the uncertainty I carry with me in a brain turned wild, drunk with death and destruction.

❧

IN ANTICIPATION OF a large harvest from our first garden, Joyce and I decided to buy the freezer of our dreams. It was large enough to store quantities of our homegrown vegetables, as well as the meat we bought on sale.

The side door into the basement was the only entry we could use. We carefully measured the door width before we went freezer shopping. Finding the perfect freezer was not difficult. It was long but not overly wide, and very deep. We found one that appeared to fit through the basement door. It was a freezer to hold a lot of food.

The basement door is narrower than a regular exterior door, but that was not the only problem. When you open the side door, there is a stairway going to the kitchen on the left and on the right a stairway going down to a low-ceilinged, concrete-floor basement. Each passage is narrow, especially the one going to the kitchen because there are walls on both sides. The stairway to the basement is more open and provides some wiggle room.

When delivery day came, we learned measuring alone does not tell the story, especially when it is necessary to make a slight turn with a large object going down a narrow stairway with little wiggle room and a low ceiling. Two men brought the big metal box. They were experienced in the artful ways of maneuvering large objects into small basements. With much sweat and careful movement they managed to get the freezer into the basement without a scratch.

As soon as the new freezer was cold, we stocked up. I made a quick harvest of broccoli, one of our best crops as it turned out, as long as it was cut young. Later, roasts and other hunks of bloody-looking meat found their way into the cold box, along with our own sweet corn, tomatoes and other vegetables. It proved to be a handy way to provide cheap food, but it took a lot of discipline and work. Screening the newspaper food pages was a chore and locating the little places with the best prices was often difficult. Over time we found ourselves heading to the nearest supermarket and the freezer was left behind to make lovely white fuzzy ice and keep the stuff in there cold.

Twenty-five years later we moved the freezer to the farm for Francesco to use. Several frozen broccoli stems were at the bottom when I cleared it before the move. I was reluctant to eat any of it after all these years.

It was just as hard to get the freezer out of the basement as it was to move it in, but it went up the long concrete walk into the barn without a hitch.

Hot cloudless blue sky days of summer settle in to choke us day and night. Even with the windows open and the fans running, we soak the sheets at night. The smell of sulfur permeates the air.

We were lucky to have two cherry trees in the backyard. One along the fence appeared to be from the original orchard out of which the development was carved. The dark, rough bark of the tree absorbed the wire fence along the property line, creating a permanent joint between the living and the dead. It was so thick you couldn't animate your fingers around its tempestuous body.

The cherries were sweet with an undercurrent of sourness. They were still plentiful and fell with abandon in the late spring. They were a magnet for birds, and by early summer the ground nearest the tree was littered with rotting cherries favored by fierce, mean yellow jackets nervously zipping around the fallen fruit.

The second tree was about ten feet from the old beauty and close to our house. It appeared to be much younger and we guessed it was self-sown from the mother tree close by. It was little more than a whip and it was growing well. I left it when we cleaned the backyard of other trees.

My tearful pen scribbles a new mark on white paper. I can see memory burning in the bright lights speeding through my midnight brain.

I still carry with me the memory of sitting in the movie theater in Eldora, Iowa, in summers of long ago. The darkness hugged me and the seats were soft and red. The show always started with a cowboy serial in which the hero galloped over a cliff to his death. To my surprise, the serial next week begins with the same cowboy galloping away from the cliff, forgetting his death. For many years, I believed this was the way death came, a game of hide and seek that allowed us to live forever if we were careful.

The sewer spits into the street with the power of its stink. Beauty is everywhere.

My introduction to Mr. Dyer, my neighbor two doors down on our side of Ivy Street, came accidentally one early spring morning soon after we moved into our house. I skipped down the front steps and picked up the paper. I took a walk around the front yard.

I looked down the street at the rows of cars. It was then I saw an old man walking on the sloping metal roof. I walked over to see what was going on and to introduce myself. I decided not to shout at the man balancing on the roof. I was afraid my noise might cause him to lose his balance.

The old man continued his inspection of the roof. He finally looked my way and waved and at the same time began to gingerly negotiate the slippery roof toward the ladder.

I introduced myself as he climbed down the ladder, and he told me his name but it was so unusual I immediately forgot the first part. From then on I always called him Mr. Dyer, out of respect and forgetfulness. He called me Tom, as did everybody else.

He showed me around his yard, full of spring-blooming flowers. He asked me if I liked gardening and flowers. I did and he was already aware of the cleanup job I did behind the house. He watched me hack at the old weeds and clear my backyard.

Mr. Dyer showed me around his backyard. He had a fine little garage with a late-model car but it was too large for the sixty-year-old garage. His grass was his pride. It was the finest, most weed-free grass I ever saw outside a country club. We stopped at a massive bed of daylilies with their wide, fresh green leaves.

Do you like daylilies? he asked.

Of course I did. My father and mother nurtured me on wild daylilies. The old man went to his basement and brought out a shovel and began digging.

I want you to have some of my daylilies, he said. They need to be separated anyway.

He dug a dozen from different spots in his backyard and I took them home. I planted the daylilies where he could see them poking their heads above my spring garden.

Over the years, Joyce and I became friends with Mr. Dyer and his wife, Myrty. It was not the kind of friendship where everything is exposed; theirs was a generation of secrets held close. There were times when Mr. Dyer was loquacious, but it was always transparent and to the point.

It wasn't until he died, and then quiet Myrty passed on, that the small secrets they hid from the world, and shared with each other, were revealed. We knew none of this until the Dyer's house was offered for sale. I saw the inside of the old house, built about the same time as ours, for the first time. Even its old furniture still sparkled.

There was a large piano in the room next to the old kitchen. Upstairs the bedrooms were spotless. In the drawers there were the clothes in which the Dyers lived, much of it pinchpenny, fresh with patches carefully sown, covering rents on almost every garment. Drawers were stuffed with carefully folded, much-darned socks and underwear. The closets hung full with patched trousers, and shirts.

In the basement, everything was well scrubbed. Although it was probably as wet as ours after a rain, it sparkled like new. Even here the old virtue of saving everything was seen in the many canning jars neatly stacked for next year's garden harvest.

Mr. Dyer delighted in telling stories about his childhood. He grew up on a farm twenty miles from what was to become Arlington, and he took a train to school in Washington, D.C., every morning. He loved to tell stories of the hardships his farming family overcame.

In his working life, Mr. Dyer was an auto mechanic, but it was his love of flowers, especially daylilies, I will remember most. Mr. and Mrs. Dyer were a kindly couple, reminders of another time, the time of my grandparents, when hard work was all there was.

In winter, birds circle in large flocks searching for something they lost when food was plentiful and the grass was green.

❋

W HEN I WAS a child, I looked forward to hometown Iowa trips. I was excited to go to Eldora because my grandparents were there. These were barely known people I saw once a year, my grandfather and mother DeBaggio on my father's side and Grandma Davis on my mother's.

I loved staying at Grandma Davis's. She had a large house with four bedrooms upstairs and downstairs there was a large room with books, magazines and something she called a stereopticon. It was a primitive device to capture a moment in time in three dimensions.

Soon after I was diagnosed with Alzheimer's, I began to see a series of still pictures after I shut my eyes to go to sleep at night.

Several years later I realized the images I saw as I went to sleep resembled the kind Grandma Davis showed me. The images I saw resembled old snapshots from yesteryear's three-dimensional stereopticon, except they were flat and two-dimensional.

Until recently, I thought these images were presented to me as they would be if they were hung on a wall and I looked them in the eye. Now I see the images from a position on the ground looking up at them. The images I see when I go to sleep in the dark are the memories held in my brain for so many forgotten years.

Now, weakened by Alzheimer's, memories leak through holes in my brain, giving me one last glimpse of who I was and where I went, a last picture show.

A SMALL BLACK dog was in my teenage life, but not until I married Joyce did I hug the pleasure of cats. Our early days together with cats were not memorable. We can remember neither cat's name, only that one died of cancer when Francesco was highchair size, and a second ran away. It wasn't until we moved to Ivy Street that we had a proper place to entertain cats. Now the house is filled with cats and their memories.

Our first cats in the house on Ivy Street came to us through a classified ad. Joyce spotted an advertisement for a pair of felines, littermates in fact. The cats were given up because of a baby and we picked up the cats and hurried home. There was some event that afternoon, perhaps a school function, and we took the box with our two young cats, opened it in the house and then absconded for a few hours. When we returned the cats had vanished. We speculated about how they escaped from our locked house. We looked everywhere up, down and under. They were gone and a mystery. About the third day, they showed up, playful and hungry. After fifteen years, they died a few days apart.

Replacing any cat is difficult, but Joyce ran into a friend at the Torpedo Factory whose mixed-breed cat delivered an overflow of kittens. He brought some of the little ones to work and Joyce was smitten with one and brought her home. This is the way we found Sabina.

I thought one cat was enough but before long a waiter at one of our favorite restaurants told us he saved several cats abandoned by their mother in the basement of an apartment house. The cats nearly drowned in a flood, but the waiter's watchful eye and concern brought them out. We took one of these glossy black kittens and called her Una.

In our living room, there is a large photograph of a cat, looking straight into your eyes from half darkness. It is not a shy cat but a steady, sweet animal. The photo is of a cat Francesco left with us when he moved to California to chase his dreams. The cat was named Nifty, and one day his insistent desire to run wild took him through our backyard and that of our neighbor and into the street where a car hit him.

I learned of the hit and run from a man who came to the house while I was eating lunch. I ran to Irving Street with fear trembling my body. I could not have run fast enough to save Nifty. There was no life left in him. I picked up his lifeless body carefully and carried him home through a veil of tears. Nifty's wild, wandering days were over.

We had cats of our own when Nifty was around and that was part of the reason Francesco's cat was unhappy to be in our house and wanted so badly to be outside. Cats are territorial and adjustment is not a word many cats understand. Our two cats were littermates and grew up with us. They considered Nifty an interloper and treated her accordingly.

I awoke this morning with a strong feeling I am not going to die of Alzheimer's. It was the first time in almost two years I felt normal and I no longer imagined myself a walking time bomb.

In time I realized growing plants was more than a way to produce family food; it could be a way of living, and a business. I began to haunt the Library of Congress, spending long hours huddled with books on plants and plant growing. I bought subscriptions to the few professional magazines that were available and devoured them on arrival. I was becoming a farmer without a farm or an acre of ground to cultivate.

My reading sent me down a traditional path to the country. No sissy backyard could accommodate a working farm. Trapped in a backyard, I saw claustrophobia destroying my dreams.

One fine fall day, Joyce and I piled in the car for a drive to the country while Francesco was at school. We headed for Loudoun County, a wide, long, scantily populated place, too far out at the time to interest developers.

The first afternoon trip encouraged me and I began to watch the newspapers for property sales. We took trips into the country to buy brightly colored fresh apples, and enjoyed detours to look at flat land for sale. By then my dream, cultivated by my reading, had begun to fasten on blueberries as the crop to grow. A visit to a small, lush blueberry farm on the way to the country place of Joyce's father grabbed me, loading my dream with personal exposure.

Our visits to Loudoun County increased and one day I fell in love with a flat piece of twelve acres. It was surrounded by larger farms and on a macadam road. A long dirt lane bordered one side of the property. There was open, grassy land for as far as we could see. Across the macadam road was a large working farm and in fall it was full of drying corn stalks, as was the large farm on a hill we could see to the west. It didn't take long to fall in love with it and it was soon ours, thanks to money left when my mother died.

We had an empty square of land and we rented it to a local farmer on a yearly basis. The lonely Loudoun dream of a blueberry farm soaked up sun, rain and snow. We lacked the nerve to grab the dream because I lacked the ability to fall in love with it.

In a few years, we had a call from another local farmer who wanted to buy my dream. It was too early to give up the dream, but over several years the eager farmer courted us with visits and slabs of beef from his cattle, brought to us personally, along with a little sales pitch. Finally we sold it to him for more than what we paid, and used the money, eventually, to finance a large greenhouse in our backyard. I realized what Joyce knew all along; the acreage was a trap of loneliness. It was a place so foreign to us we could never learn the language it spoke.

Everywhere I walk on the streets near my house I see destruction of the familiar, the precursor of new high-rise buildings for business and living. What had been snug to the ground has taken off into the unfamiliar air. The human scale is being bullied into extinction.

Mrs. Peeks lived opposite Mr. Dyer. I got to know her soon after we moved into the house on Ivy Street. In many ways she was the opposite of the ultraclean Dyers.

She lived in a small house, typical of those built in the early part of the nineteenth century. It sat close to the street, as did all the houses at the head of the narrow little street. There was a generous front porch with heavy, round pillars painted white. Upstairs there were dormers allowing air to cool the torrid summer heat. An addition was stuck on the back of the house for an additional bedroom. There were four little rooms on the first floor, including a kitchen. The backyard was heavily shaded by large abandoned trees. In fall, tan piles of crisp leaves blew into piles covering grass and earth.

Mrs. Peeks's husband was a former military man. I spoke to him a few times but he had little to say, in contrast with his voluble wife; I never knew his name. He was a smoker and Mrs. Peeks could not abide smoke in the house. Her husband was a fixture on the front porch, sitting in a chair puffing morning, noon and night, no matter the day or the weather.

For a while, I worked at Kostos art store in Georgetown, a historical site stuffed with the Washington upper class and clumsy brick sidewalks. I took Mrs. Pecks to work every morning a few blocks from where I worked. She was a seamstress with a big paper bag full of the work she had done the night before. It was a hard, long day for her, but she never complained. When her husband died she continued to sweep the walk in front of her house as well as the houses on each side of her.

It was through Mrs. Peeks I got to know Mr. King, an old crippled man who took care of her grass and shrubs and performed odd jobs for her as needed. After he died, Mrs. Peeks called on me for help with the grass, and especially when her basement flooded, as it did frequently in the spring.

The basement was unlike anything I ever saw. It was accessed from an outside door, greeted by a steep board stairs. Only half of the area under the house was used. On one side I could see thick, red clay just as it was when the house was built. The other half was dug deep, well over my head, and it had a concrete floor and eventually a sump pump to automatically suck water out of the basement into her side yard.

There were many things I did not know about Mrs. Peeks, some of which were unearthed when she reluctantly went into a nearby nursing home. I knew she was not feeding herself well but I hadn't realized how much she had let go. When the house was cleaned prior to selling it, I discovered she threw nothing away and her once delightful living room was reduced to a slender little winding path through a hodgepodge of trash. Several years of the *Washington Post* were carefully stored in a vacant bedroom. There were high piles of unwashed pots and pans in the kitchen. The end was so different, the house so still, secrets scattered in abandon, spilling over the little front yard in sad profusion.

AFTER HIGH SCHOOL I dropped out of the University of Arizona in two weeks, homesick and lonely in a place of blowing sand and beer drinking. Joyce studied art at the Corcoran School of Art in Washington, D.C., burnishing her love of art and carrying on with a crowd emptying beer cans to polish their studies.

I met her after those days when she warmed the art department of the Hecht Company with her art background. I bicycled the several miles it took from my house a few times and then began to walk against the evening traffic. It was easy to spot her salmon two-seater Austin Healy and she picked me up. We played this cat-and-mouse pickup game for several weeks. By then I showed her my collection of street "art" stones and bottles I discovered washed up against the sidewalks.

I moved into the Buckingham apartments, carrying with me all the clay, pottery wheel and other paraphernalia a hungry potter might need and set it up in what was intended to be a bedroom. I slept on a little daybed I brought from my parents' house. Joyce brought me a surprise housewarming gift, a naked mannikin from the Hecht Company storage room. I set it in the entrance to the apartment, where it was the first thing seen behind me when I answered the door.

Joyce was patient while I spun my wheels and dreamed, but she was not idle. Like me and many others, Joyce needed a time to dance on strings and stretch the feeling of adulthood.

All this took place during the trembling, angry days of Vietnam. I registered as required on my birthday. Several years later I moved into the little first-floor apartment. It was here I received a notice informing me I was to report for military service. It left me trembling as my emotions switched and water leaked from my eyes. I was afraid to go and afraid not to. Joyce was there the night I opened the envelope with the news. The war made both of us shiver, and I vowed not to be part of it. I considered emigrating to Canada, a haven for those running away from the draft. My father, unable to serve in World War II for health reasons, was upset when he learned what I was contemplating, but by then he must have realized he had little to say in my life. We got married and Joyce moved into the little apartment. We shared the sofa in the living room. She brought a parakeet to enliven the drab little apartment. The pottery was going full steam and I was working in an art store.

I was in the thrall of Armenian food, picked up from reading William Saroyan's books. I loved to cook and we had strange meals full of exotic flavors.

Joyce flirted with a job as an airline reservationist, a connection that helped us take on a whirlwind honeymoon of England, Scotland and Ireland. It was a rainy July that summer and a baby was beginning to move inside Joyce. We had fun sharing showers and sight-seeing on the gloomy, wet streets.

Vietnam began to recede as a constant fear. Married men with children were made exempt; I no longer had that threat hanging over me. Joyce's days as an airline reservationist ended.

When we returned, it was time to ask the tenants of the house on 26th Street to move. I bought the house with money I saved from several paperboy jobs over many young years. The tenants left reluctantly with a push from my father and we moved in, pottery, baby and what little furniture we had. Joyce's father built a beautiful hardwood table that we used in the dining room. I painted the room with abandon, creating large fish and funny people with unusual colors. These were days to roll in the grass with a baby in your arms, so beautiful it was hard to keep from crying.

While I worked at Hills Art Supplies I began to see the need for an alternative newspaper. I loved to write and I had won some minor awards in high school. I worked for a local daily newspaper when I was in high school. Now I had the opportunity to use all these skills.

I learned early it was easy to put a newspaper together, but the largest hurdle was distributing copies in a city in love with the status quo. An even greater failing was that my newspaper was way out in left field. I wanted it dearly and I was stupid. When money was short, I sold the house and moved the family into an apartment while I rented an office above a carwash in Georgetown. About the only things I got out of it were an angry wife left in the suburbs and two signatures of the Spanish painter Joan Miró, sent on a letter asking for a copy of the newspaper.

Young trees stand high, naked of leaves. Rough trunks and twisted stems lie everywhere. A calamity is at work where deer, squirrels and raccoons make tracks in the wet earth. We wait for the end of long nights and listen for the sounds of spring come alive.

By the time we kicked around Delaware and came back with a six-year-old and found a real house to call home, it was time for Joyce to take classes at Northern Virginia Community College, where she studied graphic arts, history and English.

The opening of the Arlington Art Center in an old school building not far from our house was the perfect place for a young artist to practice her craft and Joyce became a member of the print group there.

Our house was not far from the art center and Joyce often rode her bicycle, a dearly loved relic from her childhood days. It was far from new and, until it was stolen one day, I thought it worthless.

Several months later, Francesco spotted her bike in the rack at Washington-Lee High where he attended school. After an examination of the bike, school officials turned it over to Joyce. It still sits under the front porch, ready for its next adventure.

*   *   *

It's Thursday, trash collection day. Early morning smells of garbage float on sleepy-eyed breezes.

※

JOYCE AND I traveled to a friend's summer place recently. It was far into the country, in a place where Maryland met water before it was the sea. The house was modest, in a neighborhood of similar dwellings, many homemade and unique. Although the houses and the lots were small, the heavy green foliage in the understory and the tall leafy trees created a pleasant cool, green glade and dissolved urban frustration. From the back porch, the shimmering water flickered through the trees.

After some pleasantries and something to eat, we found our way down the narrow streets and over an embankment into soft sand that sucked at our shoes. The sky was wide and the water was open and glinting, and it lapped the shore, tan sand laughing with a child's noise.

This is a familiar place but I am told I have never been here. Was it in a dream I walked in this wet sand? Was this a forgotten moment of childhood? Far away the same ocean water wets the sky.

A young mother lifts her laughing, naked baby in and out of the gentle waves. Hurrying water laps firm wet sand in the afternoon as death plays in my body. Time is now quickly forgotten, and memory is gone. There is only now.

There is romance in a slow death, but like so much romance, it is not worth the trouble.

🖃

IT WAS EASIER to understand farming in a place with which I was familiar and on a scale I understood. Soon the backyard was filled with cold frames, simple wooden boxes with tops to take off when it became hot, a drawback that required constant inspection or the plants cooked. After the cold frames, I moved to small greenhouses, structures I put up myself with little trouble. Covering greenhouses became necessary with home greenhouses. The glass gaps allowed heat to escape as from a sieve. I often planned winter covering of the houses in fall when Francesco was home from college. He was also available in spring at just the right time to remove the plastic coverings to permit better ventilation. It was a way for the two of us to get together and at the same time for me to pass along information about growing plants to him, although at the time he had no discernable interest in what I was doing in the backyard.

I bought narrow glass greenhouses designed to be expanded by hooking one bay to another. Heating them with small gas or electric heaters was a winter nightmare, and I finally bought a gas heater for the only greenhouse used during winter when we were closed.

During spring and summer the houses were hot because the vents were too small to release enough hot air. This wasn't so bad for individuals who visited us to buy plants; a large covered area beside the house was set aside for sales. In summer, work life was a sweaty nightmare. The less expensive and larger hoop houses were eventually hooked to gas heaters. In summer these greenhouses were poorly cooled by noisy ventilating fans, and were often wet with condensation. With all these greenhouses, juggling space was a sore spot, and we moved plants around for best usage.

Eventually my backdoor neighbor complained to the county, alleging I had an illegal home business. I knew I was on firm ground legally, but I was cautious and hired a lawyer whose father had written the county code. A seven A.M. meeting was convened at the courthouse. I brought a slide show to explain what I was doing and what the facility looked like.

We talked for half an hour and the county officials admitted what I was doing was legal, except for the area next to the house where we sold plants in a long, narrow glass greenhouse. The upshot of the meeting was that I could use my backyard as long as the greenhouse was a certain distance from the house and from the back fence. To placate my complaining neighbor, I sold all my greenhouses to my customers and ordered a new green-house to fill the backyard. This structure, with bells and whis-tles, was constructed during the summer, finished the day before we opened for Christmas.

A dead unmourned squirrel lies in the street, car tracks visible across the flat, lifeless body. Bees and flies hover over the corpse. I look at it absentmindedly until I recognize in its death the fragility of my own life.

On top of a steel bench, under what is left of a dying crop in the greenhouse, is a carefully manicured bird's nest on top of a large pot filled with dirt. The first time I noticed it a small, sin-gle, pure white egg sat on a tiny obelisk. Within a few days another egg appeared. I was puzzled because I had yet to see an adult bird sitting on them for warmth.

Within a few more days, I met a mourning dove warming the two eggs in the makeshift lodging, where long, overgrown plants provided a thin canopy for Mom and her future offspring.

For many days, a serious, sensitive bird carefully warmed the eggs. She sat still, adjusting herself occasionally in a manner carefully calibrated to take her in a circle every twelve hours. Occasionally my movements sent her screaming from the green-house with much flapping of wings, but she always returned for sentry duty in spite of the hundred-plus temperatures during the summer days.

There is something strongly instinctual to keep the bird on the eggs even though it could easily fly away from them. Is it the same instinct that keeps me coming to the greenhouse to water the plants and pretend this is serious work?

The essentials of my life for the last twenty-five years have been dirt, herbs and time. There is still plenty of dirt and herbs left, but little time.

The monster living inside me showed itself last night, taking me on a wild ride down unfamiliar streets. It had all the hallmarks of Alzheimer's.

Sometime after midnight I awakened afraid and alone. I sat upright. The sheets were wet with my tears. My body was all messed up. I was crying and I had an erection. Out of my mouth ripped rough, hog-wallowing sounds, choking my ability to breathe. I panted rhythmically and cried uncontrollably.

Joyce came into the room in response to my screams and wrapped herself around me with all her life and bewilderment. Eventually the stranger inside me disappeared in the dark.

What remained of the frightening event were tears drying on my cheeks and Joyce's bewildered arms around me, trying to understand how a body so familiar can explode suddenly in the pyrotechnics of a brain slowly destroying itself.

This is a story of a crippled man imprisoned within himself.

The mourning dove's two perfectly white eggs matured and the chicks were clearly visible, even with the older bird sitting over them. There were times during the hot days I watched over the chicks while Mom was away hunting food. The family is silent and dressed sharply in soldier tan with dark markings. They parade stiffly at attention.

I was foolish enough to bring an offering to the new family, a large, fresh, red worm. They preferred their own way of gathering food. Instead of thanking me, Mom made use of the event to give her offspring early flight instructions and disappeared through an open ridge vent. The chicks dropped to the floor and danced hurriedly to the other end of the greenhouse. Even at their early age, they recognized fear.

I sit at my worktable and rub my hand over the hard brown wood. I try to squeeze words onto the clean white paper. I cannot spill the words hiding in my brain.

A little bud on a healthy, moderately tall plant in the ground of the little garden along the street has turned into a large, full-bodied artichoke; the plant produced nothing last summer and was a disappointment. Instead of harvesting the three chokes produced, I left them on the plant and watched them one after the other open into large round flowers filled with hundreds of beautiful short blue hairs. It has turned the garden into a stunning showplace.

The baby mourning doves have begun to learn to fly. They are trying to use their wings but they don't seem to have any notion of how to stop or land. Mom is around once in a while and the three of them, looking almost all the same size, stand in a group, motionless on the greenhouse bench.

When the young birds take off, they smash head first into the greenhouse walls. If the walls weren't so clear, the birds might understand they are inside. Mom doesn't seem bothered by her offspring's pratfalls. They have to learn the hard way.

The young birds swoop with the joy of being young with two fine wings flying on subtle air currents. They are young students learning the most important lessons of their new lives as they smash into the see-through walls of the greenhouse.

After they have practiced for a week in the greenhouse,

Mom leaves her babies. Soon after, one of the young mourning doves disappears. The remaining dove, an unsure swimmer in the air currents, keeps smashing into the walls. Eventually, he finds his way out and into the world.

This is a county fair of the mind.

～

FRANCESCO AND I were prepared for the trip to nowhere and we were on our way to the airport. We weren't really going nowhere; we were going to Ohio. All places about which I know little are nowhere until I get there and find life in a different setting.

We waited in Washington National Airport long after the plane was scheduled to depart. Eventually the airplane arrived and we found our seats. We were uncomfortably pushed up against the cockpit. It was the first time I looked into a cockpit. It was a very small space. The pilot and the copilot scrunched into a space so small they crawled on all fours to get in or out.

Before we took off, the pilot crawled out of the cockpit and addressed the passengers. All the seats were filled. The pilot began walking up and down the aisle apologizing for the lack of space and the delayed takeoff. When he was through he crawled into the cockpit and we took off. It was the most unusual thing I ever encountered on an airliner, and I shouted my thanks to him through the open door.

The little plane taxied out on the runway and soon took off. The plane hung in the sky as if it were attached to clouds. Inside knees bent in to the steel wall of the cockpit and vibrations made our bodies hum. We sailed through the air with our seat belts fastened and we knew we sat on a flotation cushion.

I watched the pilot through the open door. The noise was steady and my ears were uncomfortable. I saw the pilots talking but the noise was so loud I could not hear their words.

I looked out the little window while Francesco settled down with his book. We were flying through Great Lakes clouds with a cold wind blowing down from Canada. The plane bounced around and the pilot made adjustments and folded his arms, looking straight into the sun with his powerful sunglasses. Under us the thick clouds became thin lines of a white stream. Over the pilots shoulder the ice floes were breaking up.

The fish in the pond
follow one another
circling back and forth.
They make a sucking sound
cleaning stones of food
at water's edge.
The clouds blow away.

AUGUST 26, 1992

Dear Linda,

It was clear the night in July I saw the black hole in you that death brings, the death of someone near and valuable. It is something I should have recognized immediately because of Joyce's own daily struggle to come to terms with the death of her father.

I lost my parents many years ago. Politics, culture and religion grew to divide me from them in an agonizing battle of wills, and I remember their deaths without tears or grief. I saw their pain as death drew near and I did not have the courage to acknowledge my grief when they died. The black holes left by their deaths four years apart remained with me many years later.

This is nothing in the twinkling cosmos, but it is what is left to the living. I wanted to let you know I looked inside you that hot July day and saw this dark, turbulent thing inside you. It will feel raw and uncomfortable for a long time, but it will become a source of strength, too.

During the early days I learned to accept dirt and long hours. Rising early was ingrained in me from my childhood days of delivering newspapers before leaving for school. There was a little greenhouse in back and a lean-to beside the house where we sold the plants grown in the backyard. In the early days, I dreamed of having a plant business at home that was open year-round.

The first year was a hard tryout, even though there had been several earlier attempts and many trips to the Library of Congress for education. A small, inexpensive glass greenhouse was purchased. Seeds were bought and carefully sown in rows in open flats. I had no customer mailing list so I put small ads in the *Washington Post*. I also placed a sign on 10th Street. A trickle of interest turned at Ivy Street and stopped at the first house where the driveway was littered with plants. These were days when herbs were not widely available and were of little interest to gardeners. I was lucky to have few customers because I made many mistakes. Many of the customers gave me advice and I followed some of it and forgot the rest. There was a lot for me to know.

Early in the first summer I learned more than I expected. As June began, the heat soared. There was no sign of rain and the ground became parched, cracking with thirst. I was lucky to have a single customer. I waited under what shade was available under the cherry tree in the back or from the front porch. This kind of waiting is full of anxiety.

July came and the sun got hotter as the days lengthened. Salty sweat ran in rivulets from my brow to my feet. I couldn't keep dry. The county instituted water restrictions, banning water use outdoors and restricting its use inside (flush your toilet once a day). I paid no attention to the restrictions and watered morning and night to keep from losing my stock of new transplants. I often spent three or four hours watering each day to save my plants.

While the heat intensified I was lucky to have a customer or two before noon. At noon there might be a few military people who inhabited nearby office buildings. I ate alone under the cherry tree where I could keep an eye on the lean-to and the plants. It was too hot to stay in the stifling hoop house and I spent afternoons on the porch reading until my eyes were weary and I pined for human conversation. It was the most intensive period of loneliness I ever encountered because I was anchored to the spot.

As a day came to an end, I looked forward to at least one customer, but there were often none. In the late afternoon neighbors returned from work and we often had pleasant conversations from the front steps. One day the school superintendent came by and chatted with me for a while. He lived nearby and had wide interests. The next day he came again. He stopped almost every day and we chatted. I have always been thankful for those wonderful talks that broke the melancholy of that long hot summer when reading stung my eyes. After that summer, I shrank the period of selling herbs to three and a half months beginning in mid-March, something complaining customers still don't understand.

I made it though that tough summer and before long there were more little greenhouses. I found it necessary to begin to hire part-time workers in the spring. It was a tricky business and at first there were many applicants. As years went by, the number of people looking for part-time work in the greenhouse dwindled and I sometimes took anyone interested, frequently with unhappy results.

The days began at five A.M., just enough time to breakfast and finish chores so I was ready for the first employee to arrive at seven. I spent three to four hours watering every morning in spring. There was little difference between the house where I lived with Joyce and the greenhouse out back where I worked with several people who worked three to four months in spring. Outside that short time, I had plenty to do but I needed help.

After closing at six each evening, I ate dinner and went back to work, this time sowing seed. Seed sowing was staggered so I didn't have all the plants we sold at one time. The plants were always fresher that way.

Along with the heat came bugs, something of a problem, especially as the summer progressed. Spraying was done two to three times a week depending on the time of year. It was necessary to wear special clothes and a face mask. Even long after dark, it was so hot inside the special spraying suits that water ran down my body and I often had to dump sweat water out of my shoes. By eleven P.M. I usually dropped into bed until morning when it started all over again, no matter the day of the week.

How I did it for nearly twenty-five years, I'll never know. Perhaps it was the excitement of being free of a boss and in charge of my life. It could have been the excitement of being on the edge of an exciting new world with roots centuries old. Maybe it was that there was nothing else I'd rather have done.

Every minute I breathe I am on the edge of tears.

The mythic limestone stream, bubbling cold and clear from mysterious underground sources, captured my imagination the first time I saw Mossy Creek. I didn't even take my rod from its tube.

I anticipated difficulty fishing the narrow, grassy waters and fast-moving currents cutting through high banks molded from rough pastureland. A city boy, I did not anticipate the deep silence of the bright sky and the pasture surrounded by gray, grassy hummocks. Instead of fishing, I walked around the cows

and watched their tails swish as they bathed in the legendary
waters.

The high tangles of weeds full of grasshoppers whispered in
the breeze, and I became mesmerized by the water and the landscape. It was easier to enjoy the surroundings than to test my
skills against the water's reputation for wise, elusive brown
trout, a distinction made palpable this late summer day by the
silence around me and the absence of other anglers.

The drive to Mossy was long and to spend no time fishing
seemed to waste the day in idleness, which was unlike me.
Slowly, I came to understand I sought not fish, but a romantic
vision of earth, air and water. If that vision ever materialized, it
vaporized when I slipped on a fresh cow pie and a couple of
cows eyed me menacingly. Farm boys feel at home here, but I
am a creature of the manicured suburban utopias that mush-
roomed on the edge of cities during the fifties and I was bewildered by the beauty and stubbornness of this rolling land.

I didn't need a romantic angling vision to bring me back to
Mossy. I hired a teacher to initiate me into the secrets of spring
creek fishing. The guru was Harry Murray, the pharmacist, author and clairvoyant of Virginia Blue Ridge Mountain fishing.

I arrived before Harry, after a short tutorial held in town.
While I waited, I went to the edge of the little dirt parking area
above the creek. The big brown I saw earlier on my previous
trip was gone. I remembered how it rose slowly through the
shallow water to gulp ants with a steady rhythm and then, suddenly, for no imaginable reason, darted under a mossy island.
The many tippets tangled in the branches above the brown's
feeding station gave witness to the frustration of many anglers. I
did not realize then how rare and unusual was the sight of such
a fish.

That first day Harry lent me his magical nine-foot Scott 4-
weight for which he ordered two tips after an angling accident
in Montana decommissioned it. He pointed and I side-armed a

cast in the direction his finger suggested. The big hopper landed and there was an immediate splash as a fourteen-inch brown dashed for it. The fish discovered the phony, tasteless body before I set the hook. Harry gave me a frustrated but kindly look, imparted some wisdom, and moved on to his next student.

I tired of beating the water and started walking downstream. There is a delightful spot where the stream turns left under the shade of tall, old trees that line a high bank. The trees offered me shade and I sat for a moment to rest. As my eyes searched the water, I saw a pod of several dozen fish eagerly taking food from the current. I tied on a little gold ribbed hare's ear, swung my line in a long curve and let the current drift the fly through the cluster of eight-inch browns. One after another that afternoon they jumped on the little hook. Was it the rod, or the beautiful October day? I cared not. The pleasure of catching fish until you're so tired you don't want to catch more has been rare in my experience.

This is my long good-bye.

I looked forward to my next visit to Mossy with great anticipation, but I didn't return until the following August. I first went upstream, only a hundred yards from the parking area. Browns were dimpling the late afternoon water with their rises. My offerings failed to tempt them and discouragement nestled in the corners of my mind. A day of dry hopes, the crash of wind and temperature in the upper atmosphere—all often produce the lightning of sudden illumination. I thought such angling revelations might be encouraged by returning to the hole below the mound of trees where Mossy took a left turn.

From above, looking through the water, I saw nothing but the stony bottom. I crept along the narrow path, now at mid-summer bordered with thick, dense, head-high weeds. There, next to a stone outcropping, a sixteen-inch brown snacked. I headed down the path to get into position when suddenly the rest of the world became illuminated in a loud commotion behind me. The hoofs of a herd of cows pounded the dry, yellow clay path into fine dust as they galloped toward me like an out-of-control train.

There was only one way out, and I began to run along the narrow footpath away from the thundering hoofs, down the bank toward the turnstile crossing, a sturdy barbed-wire fence about thirty yards distant. I sprinted with the breathless fear of a city boy and made it over the fence with the massive lead bovine inches from my back.

There was no gloating in my glance as I panted and looked back at the decidedly unfriendly cows milling around the fence shouting menacing moos at me. I sauntered forty yards downstream pretending to resume my fishing. In a few minutes, I looked back upstream where I intended to begin my approach toward the feeding trout. I saw the huge black and white lead cow that led the stampede standing in the mud as the water swirled over its hooves. From my vantage point, the cow appeared to be waving its tail at me in a bovine gesture of contempt. I fished no more that day. I needed time to plan the best route back to my car without disturbing the cows in the pasture.

Report to Colleen A. Blanchfield, M.D.

OCTOBER 13, 2000

In the last three weeks, I have lost much of my ability to multiply and add numbers, especially numbers containing 7s. What is not used now seems to decay quickly.

Word comprehension is becoming more difficult but most of the time by studying the word I eventually recognize it. Some common words, familiar for years, seem new to me.

Language use is also more difficult. There are more instances of temporary word loss. When this happens I try to describe the word's meaning or appearance to my companion (often Joyce), hoping they will recognize the word for me. Sentences I write sometimes stop before the finish line. I knew where the sentence was bound but part of it fell over a cliff before I could type it. I sit in wonderment and anger, unable to fill the space where the runaway sentence formed and flashed away.

When I close my eyes at night white klieg lights sweep my shut eyes with a blinding brilliance. The light is steady and pointed directly at me, illuminating an emptiness as large as a desert. I wonder whether this bright white light is searching for something or someone who is lost.

My cat Sabina continues to guard me each night from a place on my bed, as she has since the word Alzheimer's entered my vocabulary.

A COUPLE OF months after the mourning doves left the greenhouse, one returned. I recognized the dove easily. It was the bird that had slammed into the walls of the greenhouse. It was nice to see him return for a little remembrance tour.

IN THOSE EARLY days of hunger and youth, I was a man who, spring and fall, had the blade of a spade and the prongs of a fork buried in the soil, creating a more fecund earth. I loved digging, the act of it and the look of it. Sometimes I thought the newly turned earth looked so pretty after leveling it into a soft, smooth surface I hesitated to spoil it with plants.

Earth, soft earth, that is something lovely and useful and, in my limited experience, something hard to find. Gardeners are fortunate. From East to West and from North to South, farmers have to live with the acres given them. Gardeners, on the other hand, can create a verdant paradise on the few square feet they buy, rent or beg.

I took the spading fork with the thick, square tines and began the arduous task of turning and loosening the soil to a depth of about twelve inches. I was careful to smash the clods—and there were many—into dust and remove the stones. After I turned the area and raked it level, I stood back to judge the work and wipe sweat from my face and neck. The work would have been easier if the soil were sandy, but I knew I was to amend it with first class soil so it would hold water necessary for the plants to flourish.

Soon I was hauling loads of compost, that crumbly, dark mixture of manure, earth and decomposed leaves and vegetable scraps, and dumping it on the newly turned soil. The perennial herbs I planned to plant here would survive for many years and during that time I wanted to disturb the plants' roots as little as possible. I had one chance to make it right. Load after load of humus was dumped until I could rake out a level frosting of compost about five inches thick. When I ran out of the home-made compost, I substituted dampened sphagnum peat or dried manure. This was the best way to condition the soil so it contained plentiful air pockets the roots could use to breath.

I raked the top level smooth and with my garden fork began to thoroughly mix everything together, top to bottom. When I finished, I raked the edges toward the center of the bed and placed rot-proof two-by-eights around the perimeter to give the area an architectural character and to prevent water runoff. I finished by dusting the surface with lime and 5-10-5 fertilizer. I aimed for a pH of 6.5 for the garden.

Seeds and a long, nervous wait were necessary while germination began to secretly expand in the dark earth until one day skinny reeds pushed through the soil to announce spring's birth.

❊

Some mornings, after I take two Exelon tablets, I float away on a tranquil sea. It is an unwelcome feeling and I cannot work efficiently until early afternoon. I mentioned the condition to Dr. Blanchfield and she immediately cut my Exelon dose in half and began Aricept again, one tablet at night.

Gone are the days of swaggering youth. I have reached an age at which I can see my mortality reflected in the daily obit page.

My daily walk at dawn takes me along a path made familiar by many years of use. I take the sidewalk along Wilson Boulevard toward Ballston, turn right on Glebe Road, and return home via Fairfax Drive. My many steps equal about three miles and follow an everyday sameness. For me, the subtle changes of the familiar sights provide an avenue from which to inspect the present and reflect on the past.

When I pass Dunkin' Donuts early in my morning sojourn, I see the building, but I also see what used to be there: the black, flat asphalt parking lot used by Edmonds' Ford, formerly at the corner of 10th and Wilson and now occupied by Arlington Auto Care.

As I pass Mario's Pizza, I remember the smell and wonder of it when it first opened. I worked as a kid reporter after school at the *Northern Virginia Sun* in those high school days. The newspaper was where Arlington-Pentagon Cleaners is now, across the street from Mario's. It was at the *Sun,* working for 25 cents a column inch, that I tripped on several of my earliest moral dilemmas, and realized the power of the written word.

Farther along, across from the Arlington Art Center, sterile asphalt supports used cars where once stood an old tavern, legendary as much for the smell of its ancient beer-stained floor as it was historic.

What is now called Ballston has a rich lode of memory for me. I recall as a youth traveling down Wilson Boulevard in a bus. I saw dust rising above a solid wooden fence there. I turned to my father for an explanation and he told me it was a sign the Washington Redskins were scrimmaging on what was then their practice field.

My most important memories of this piece of earth, near the intersection of Wilson Boulevard and Glebe Road, came long after the Redskins left, unseated by the Hecht Company department store. Passing Hecht's releases strong, sweet memories. It was in this fortress-like building I first met Joyce behind the art supply counter. I befuddled her with strange, lonesome stories, and then talked her into marrying me.

An open place across Glebe Road from the Hecht Company also calls forth special memories. It once housed an art supply store called Hill's in which I spent several years selling and making picture frames. Every morning I glance at where it once stood and my memory promptly recalls incidents from that time, so full of promise and happiness, common to all those newly married with a baby. It was also a time of shadowy anxiety on the cusp of the country's most rending modern moment, the Vietnam War. This area is the closest to a holy shrine of any place along my route.

In recent months, I have become accustomed to the sudden sepulchral shadows of bulldozers that appear innocently one morning and, by the next day, stand naked beside a pile of rubble.

My early-morning walks may not have the thrill of a daybreak stroll through Rome, where it appears nothing is thrown away and everything remains as it has been for centuries, but the daily hike is more than a stroll down memory lane. I have come to realize my morning constitutional holds important remnants of comfort, anger, inquiry, wonder, bewilderment and friendship. My walks offer all the things necessary for intelligent life.

As my personal landmarks have begun to disappear, I have awakened to an unsettling side of the American character. Instead of preserving the mundane and ordinary from a past we constantly demolish it, destroying the keys to our own and society's rich past and to an understanding of the present. The habitat of twentieth century America, polished by its residents with laughter and hardship, has begun to shift constantly, leaving an uncertainty with a disturbing power to destabilize our lives.

An artifact is sometimes necessary to light a long hidden memory. When all the artifacts disappear, memories lie dormant in a place where the past cannot be examined with the fresh eye of the present. Memory, which others may call history, has the power to nourish our inner lives, and without it much is lost to the present and to the future. Whether the absence of these personal landmarks and their memories is a fatal affliction remains to be tested.

The air rumbles as the airliner splits the clouds on its ascent. A shower of jasmine floats through the night air.

The cats bedded in informal boxes or floating on soft chairs pretend sleep, their slit-eyes watch my every move and turn of the page. I think they have the ability to take my pulse from afar. They are careful watchmen, these doctors without portfolio, knowing everything, revealing nothing.

IN THE MIDST of the celebration of the end of World War II, two natural phenomena, typical of a child's world, seduced me with their wonders.

First came a fondness for digging in dirt and, soon after, I became attracted to water, an element that might have appealed to me initially had I not associated it with baths, something I preferred to avoid. I learned at war's end that water, in the form of rain, left delightful puddles in which to splash and play. At this early age water and dirt were firmly joined in my pantheon of pleasures. More serious from my parents' point of view, I showed up to dinner with muddy clothes every night. Sometimes dreams clash with other's standards.

The puddle of which I was so fond was at the foot of North Nicholas Street where the paving gave way to yellow dirt just before crossing a foamy little creek. Other temporarily wet places sprang to life in the aftermath of summer thunderstorms, where paper boats floated gaily on an imagined sea. Of all these transient puddles I loved most the muddy pool at the entrance to Mr. Turner's property. It was here that my love of small wet places was created.

As a teenager, I discovered a way to continue my involvement with puddles without juvenile embarrassment. I built a fish pool in the corner of a backyard patio my father made. This pool, with sloping sides of concrete, was home to goldfish and a water lily. Soon, however, my interest in dirt, specifically clay with which to make pottery, overcame my love of water and the little patio pool went dry. Then came years of wandering and journalism.

❁

THIS BOOK IS full of the thoughts I have in the pure innocence of early morning when I turn east and face the warm, soft sun. There is a freshness and purity that inhabits mornings, and some people call it hope. Whatever it is, it penetrates the mind as it awakes and orders its memories. It is easy to spin elaborate conceits in the light of a beautiful morning and to believe all thought is washed clean of sophistry and is good and true. By nightfall, those morning thoughts often appear silly and surreal, but it is good to recall them because they are part of the day's reality. The conflict between the tender, hopeful glow of the morning and the anxiety of the hard, dark evening is healed in the garden, where opposites are resolved in activity delighting mind and body.

Gardening encompasses the joys and sorrows of all life in a few months—birth, energy, fruitfulness, seriousness, laughter, death, and sometimes the surprise of resurrection. A spade in the earth is not a heavy responsibility, but gardening is a worthwhile endeavor and teaches much about the renewal of life, if you are open to it.

"The love of dirt is among the earliest of passions, as it is the latest," Charles Dudley Warner said in his long-lost book, *My Summer in a Garden*. "Muddies gratify one of our first and best instincts. So long as we are dirty, we are pure."

I am an earnest fellow—too much so perhaps for my own good—but that thought stuck with me and nourished my enthusiasm. It is an idea I sanctioned long before I read it and appeals to folks like me. To us romantics who spend much time alone in the garden or in silent rooms, it is possible these special experiences give our lives a quirky vision that leads to the acceptance of some pretty strange stuff.

I live now hovering gently between awareness and emptiness.

Joyce and I went on buying sprees after I was diagnosed with Alzheimer's. I bought fishing gear I will never use. She outfitted herself after years of holding back. I had dreams I knew were blasted.

At first I thought the buying sprees were initiated to hide the secrets pulling me apart. Now I realize it was probably an effort to renew our lives together by starting over again as if none of this happened, coloring my last days with joy while I slowly slip away.

※

As THE FIRST year on Ivy Street came to an end, I began to have dreams of pools again. I chose a place in the backyard where a disreputable garage stood. I dug a hole, shaped the inside with cement, filled it with water, and imagined how the garden around it was going to look. My neighbor looked over the back fence. Her face told me she thought I was crazy.

Eventually this pool was filled with earth, as my love affair with dirt again became ascendant, and a greenhouse went up where it had been. Instead of letting my dream of lovely water escape, I found a new place for a pool, flush up against the rear foundation and next to a high cement wall supporting the back porch. This was not a fancy pool, just a hole lined with black plastic thick enough to keep water from seeping out.

The pool was in a place to look down upon, and when the light was right I saw all the way to the bottom. While looking down on this water one night, I realized bodies of water unshackle memory and encourage romance.

A pool of water without fish or a spray of shimmering liquid activating the water's surface is without poetry or honor. To complete the pool, I purchased a dozen feeder goldfish for a dollar. Feeder fish have a sense of poverty and inevitability about them but they do not lack a certain nobility. They are small fish intended for the pleasure of larger members of their kind who will eat them. My new pool lacked big mouths and the feeders were safe. Or so I thought.

One morning I went out to feed my goldfish but the pool was empty. The missing fish became a mystery. We discussed frequently who the kidnapper might be. I bought more feeder fish almost immediately to keep the pool busy, not to tempt the fates. The next morning I arose and looked anxiously at the pool. The fish were gone, but so was the water, except for a low puddle in the middle. We dropped the idea of the neighbor's kid and substituted a raccoon.

Mysteries gnaw at mind and spirit until truth is a certainty. The solution fell to my clever son, Francesco. He set up a trip wire on the side of the house activated by a bell inside, if boy or raccoon broke it. For several nights, the bell was activated, but we saw nothing and the trip wire remained intact. Another mystery was building, but it did not last long. On the fourth night, about nine P.M. we heard a commotion in the pool and ran to the back porch to see a wet raccoon turning the corner of the house where he went under the trip wire, moving it enough to send a signal.

The raccoon was a formidable opponent. The solution was to buy a round, six-foot-wide cattle watering trough from the Sears farm supply catalog. When the truck arrived with it, we put the watering trough in the hole where the pool had been. No raccoon was going to punch holes in this new pool, although he did return once or twice to bathe (we learned several years later that he had been living in a neighbor's garage). Instead of fish we bought a little fountain statue and regularly added chlorine bleach to the water to kill the inevitable mosquito larvae.

Without fish, the pool was lifeless and boring, and one Saturday I walked to the pet store and purchased four small koi, one of the most beautiful fish species in the world. By the second year, only two of the fish had survived.

The fish changed my attitude about fish and pools. These fish were too beautiful and special to keep in a tub of water without the proper care. I began to learn something about keeping fish and what they needed. I soon purchased a large, rock-filled biological filter.

The filter increased the water quality, but it had another

influence as well. A year after the filter was installed, during spawning time, something marvelous occurred. The fish became parents, and by extension I became a grandfather to sixty or seventy fry so small I could hardly recognize them. In six months their shapes and colors made them recognizable and some individuals began to stand out. I watched them for hours as their colorful shapes darted through the water and jumped at the food as I floated it down to them. They exuded a joy in living from their watery world.

The birth of all these fish also brought some anxiety. I could see how quickly they were growing and I had seen how quickly the little eight-inch fish I purchased became twenty-inch monsters. I began to worry about what I was to do with all these fish.

Winter is moderating and warmer days are here sporadically. Wandering around the brick patio behind the house, I have fallen in love with watching the water drops leaking from the fish pool filter.

The early days were filled with false starts, sweat and loneliness. There was little need for paid employees when I started growing and selling plants from my backyard. It took several years before the need made it necessary to advertise in the *Washington Post* and hire a few part-timers.

Much of the advertising in the beginning was word of mouth and I took everybody's name and address who visited us as I built a customer list. Within a few years, I put together a catalog and mailed copies to our regular patrons.

While he lived in California, a dream took up residence in Francesco. It was a noble dream of working with his hands to nurture plants and to build beautifully landscaped, rocky pools with gently splashing waterfalls. He built several for himself and for others, and he brought his dream of fish and water gardens east with him when he returned to work with me at the nursery.

I never heard a scientist claim dreams are part of the gene pool shared by a family, and I will not offer such an assertion now. My little fish pools were much less exalted than those designed by Francesco. I asked him to build a slice of his dream in our backyard. Any hole in the ground with some liquid in it satisfied me; this is definitely not the way my son looks at water and stone.

Pools, ponds, creeks, rivers, oceans are truly foreign territory, places we can visit but in which we are unable to live. Whether these holes in the ground occur naturally or are handmade, they are places of discovery that enlarge our inner world. The creatures who reside in them live outside our atmosphere in a place with its own structure and rules, where air is replaced by water and feet become tails.

Francesco's artistic method is unique, and intuitive. Almost Zen-like, the idea for a particular pool and its form rise from his contemplation of the site. Before he began to dig, or even look at a shovel, I saw him crouch and stare intently at the spot I had chosen for the first pool. He remained in what looked like a near-trance state for many minutes, oblivious to everything around him. He was, of course, visualizing the pool and its every rock, and, perhaps, the building of each section. After several days, observing the spot, he said he was ready to begin and offered to draw me a sketch, but I told him this wasn't necessary.

Francesco's construction methods are as unusual and old-fashioned as is his method for making the perfect pool for the intended location. Arduous hard work with a shovel is his preferred digging technique. Thick rubber liners or concrete (or both together) are his usual materials. He carefully handpicks individual stones to decorate the pool's edge and mortars them together smoothly with a painter's brush, creating an artistic impression from common materials.

I watched him carefully as he worked through the heat of last summer. I realized he had a dream of dirt and water. It was not my dream, but his own, expressed in a singular way. As I observed his careful working style one afternoon, I saw moist excitement in his eyes as he labored over the exact placement of each stone around the pool's apron. In many ways, he and I are different, but our lives are animated by the inner life we call dreams.

✿

My family dreamed for centuries. A dream brought my great-grandfather to America. A dream lured my grandfather into the restaurant business, and much later he nestled into a small farm to ride horses in retirement.

My father's head was filled with many dreams and he used to reveal them over the dinner table, but his practical soul prevented him from following many of them. I saw what this did to him and vowed I would follow my dreams, no matter how impractical. Dreams are the first steps that lead to self-discovery, sometimes a very private encounter, and at other times quite public, but always beautiful in a special way making eyes glow with moisture.

Dreams are the poems our minds construct while our bodies idle, wishing for better times, if not perfection itself, something to energize its shadow. Such is the power of this dream poetry, both written and visual, that it is better to respond to the emotion or the dream immediately than it is to try to categorize it and understand it. There is plenty of time for thought later; grab at the wonder, excitement, and beauty while they are present.

*   *   *

I stretch out in the freezer and forget the hot summer sun. It is cold and dark with the lid shut but comfortable here alone. If I can only remember who I am, I can find the shelf where I belong.

Last summer my usual aches and pains lasted well beyond the end of spring rush. I found myself unexpectedly harnessed to a profound bout of melancholy. I tried to excise the pain and bury the gloom in good thoughts, but I could not rid myself of this uncommon malaise. My emotional state became so irritated I could hardly go into the garden to pick a tomato or a handful of basil. Weeding, mending fences and general cleanup were all chores I let slip.

Eventually, I fell into a meditative mood. I have lived a wickedly overworked life and my last chance to taste a little wild life is fast approaching. I decided to search the wild side for what corrective pleasures it offered.

The best way to start my own wild life was to study the birds and bees, mice and bugs sharing my square of the earth. I did not know where to begin but I was immediately attracted to the night, where identity can be easily hidden and behavior is less inhibited.

On our little patio, I spent several evenings with a family of fat, happy slugs. They turned out to be the perfect subjects to begin my study. I did not want to jump into the middle of over-active wildlife; I wanted to take it slowly and that is the slug's forte. I was not enchanted by their slothful ways, especially their eating habits. What can be said about their eagerness to drink someone's leftover beer? Nor did I care for their slime. I envied their slow, deliberate pace, however. I considered this trait one of their most valuable assets and a high point of my study.

Near the patio I decided to observe the fish in the fine, clear pool Francesco built them. While they might not meet a strict scientific definition of wildlife because they were born in captivity, they might still have the key to slow but real excitement. I had a pair of koi in an earlier pool and one reason for the new, larger pool was the amorous ways of these stately, colorful fish. There are now dozens of them. This appeared to be wild life to teach me something.

Koi are naturally acrobatic fish capable of rare displays of individuality, but they are conformists at heart, swimming together with the easy assurance of a synchronized team. Despite their sometimes inhibited character, I discovered a wild streak in them I failed to see until the week of the great jumping contest.

At first I did not know the meaning of the dead fish lying on the patio four feet from the pool. It was a large colorful koi and I inspected its body for cuts or abrasions that might have been made by a raccoon but there was no damage. I wrapped the fish and buried it in the garden.

The next morning, a second fish lay on the bricks of the patio in almost the same spot as the dead fish of the day before. The third day brought another dead fish on the patio. I began to see a deepening mystery. I sought an explanation from my books on koi and the mystery was quickly solved. Koi love to jump, the books said. I realized a jumping competition among the fish turned deadly. I immediately installed a barrier around the pool to prevent jumping fish from sailing onto the patio. There have been no more dawn encounters with dead fish. Wild life turns out to be treacherous and playful, masking a death wish.

Children are playing in an alley, young voices of joy hover around a day care troop. Hot sidewalks bake my shoes. Radios blast as a light snow falls on the empty bus.

I realized last night how Alzheimer's wrapped around me so slowly I didn't recognize it. I have deposited money in the bank for years and, for a time, every day. But last night I couldn't understand any of the procedures needed to prepare a deposit.

It came from a simple request. Francesco asked me to take a deposit to the bank. He filled out the forms for the commercial account. This was something I did for more than twenty-five years almost every day. Now I couldn't make sense of it at all.

Francesco also wanted me to write a check from my personal checking account to the business so he could pay employees. I tried to set up the computer to write a check. I couldn't understand the images on the screen. I didn't have a clue how to write the check, something I had done regularly for years. I was in tears before I asked Joyce for help and she explained everything and got the check printed.

I trembled with anger and bewilderment when I got to the bank. Some of the tellers at the bank are unaware of my mental illness and look at me with bewilderment sometimes. The bank is now one of the places I avoid if I can. It was another reminder of how far along I have walked on the path with Alzheimer's.

I am also becoming more uncertain of my body and mind. Sometimes I spend empty hours alone trying to catch air with my hands. I feel the air against the movement of my hands, but I see nothing. That is the way Alzheimer's looks.

There is a continuous hissing in my head, a sound as might be uttered by an old radiator. It is something I have learned to accept. I cannot remember when it started, perhaps when I began to take the Alzheimer's medicines. My hand is steady. No, my age is not making this buzz between my ears, nor is it whisky.

The fig tree on the south side of the house was heavy with sweet, swelling green skins, soon to be sticky ripe fruit. No one ever considered a fig tree a model for wild life and I thought that sitting under its modest height made a perfect, quiet place to rest from my studies. What a surprise lay before me.

It was a dark, warm night when I decided to pick my beautiful round figs. I grabbed a flashlight and hurried outside to begin the harvest. The fig tree is next to the house, on the south side next to the bay trees. It is a place of sun, protected from chill winter winds. I flashed my light on the fat figs and found them half eaten. I blamed the birds first, but on second thought too much had been eaten for the culprit to be a bird.

I saw many figs untouched, and about the time I took a gardener's sigh, a mouse jumped on my shoulder. It was a medium-sized gray mouse, new to the area, and it was clear he was guarding the figs from large marauders like me.

As it turned out, like most wildlife and many humans, he never finished a fig. He ate bits from several figs for several nights and then moved on to another branch. I was happy to go back to the figs boxed in my refrigerator, protected from wildlife. I didn't need a flashlight to find my figs anymore.

I looked at my left hand, as if for the first time. In the light I did not recognize the owner of these digits. The fingers were reddish with lines running up and down and crosswise. It was not a new hand or lumpy; a nice hand but surely not mine. Look at the long hairs on the back of the hand, what purpose are they? The hairy knuckles, for what purpose did the dogs make this wrinkled weeny?

Birds float above on magic currents, as my brain empties the memories keeping me alive.

The real wild life is not in Arlington, no matter how many slick watering holes are permitted to open on Clarendon's bar strip. The real wild animals, those with heft and frightful panache, are in Loudoun County. There Francesco battles a real army of groundhogs, deer, insects of both the flying and crawling persuasions, larger than nature allows in polluted areas such as

Arlington, giant wasps, and a woodlot full of poison ivy. This is just what can be outlined in mixed company. On five acres, even the grass becomes a wild, untamed force of nature.

I always try to leave the farm before nightfall. I tell Francesco I have to leave before dark to avoid the traffic jams. The truth is traffic jams occur because so many people flee the country wildlife.

The last daze is coming.

There are days filled with languid time in which a vacation attitude prevails. I thumb through magazines and investigate fishing rod catalogs when I should be working but I cannot push my dreams away long enough to begin scribbling.

I prefer to live in this make-believe world of soft air-conditioned breezes where everything is perfect and without frustration. Alone in this room, no one sees whether I am working or playing and it is easy to become someone else in this hidden place of imagination. I am a little boy again, hiding in a box, dreaming of the impossible, the unbelievable.

I pull out a fishing reel and take it apart, stroking it and admiring its shape and color, and I drift off into another world. I am streamside on Mossy Creek, kneeling in the high grass, casting to a shaded spot where the water is dream deep and slow. Suddenly the water explodes and the world is full of a large, beautiful trout, which I reel in and gently release. Sitting in my air-conditioned room my body tingles with excitement at the dream.

My piscatorial dreams are often structured by the arrival of Len and Carol Codella's *Heritage Sporting Collectibles* catalog. On the surface, it is a cheap black and white paper sales weapon. It is filled with used and new handmade bamboo fishing rods and reels. While the entries appear to be simply descriptive, they are full of heavenly poetry for a landlocked angler frustrated with unfulfilled fishing dreams.

Here is a typical entry from the summer 2000 catalog, the kind of thing that sets me off on hours of dreaming: "11536. Lancaster-R.W. 6;pr3". Baetis. 2/2. #4.2/25 oz. Medium/Fast Dry Fly. Cork Dural Ring. Antique Gold/Black. Tung Oil Impregnated. Bob Lancaster has been hand planing his meticulously built rods for more than 25 years, testing and refining his rod tapers to enhance the parabolic type of action promoted by Young. His rods not only compare favorably, but on some planes easily surpass those earlier rods. Lancaster offers a nicely made rod with an attractive Young-like appearance and a magnificent rod action for a reasonable price. That clearly makes his product a winner in our book. This rod has a strong similarity to the acclaimed Paul Young Midge, in length, line weight, appearance and casting feel. Flamed cane. Oxidized Nickel Silver Super-Z style ferrules. Tung Oil Impregnated Matte Finish. Cigar Grip. Cork seat with Knurled, Oxidized dual rings. Your chance to have the sharp, crisp and satisfying dry fly action of a finely tuned Semi-parabolic taper without paying Classic rod money for it. With labeled cloth bag, rod grip pads, and aluminum case. Brand New. $750."

Even the rod names have an allure richly etching the mind with memory: Savage River, Bighorn River, Falling Springs. Imagine how many such entries there are in a single sixty-six-page catalog and it explains why I can't get any work done and even less fishing.

It is hard to resist such a come-hither offer, and I am embarrassed to have invested when I should have hidden the catalog. Days of fishing are rare and almost always more difficult, and less rewarding, than sitting at home under an air conditioner dreaming of fly rods.

Other invitations keep me from the stream. No fish escapes

when I cast perfectly in the backyard in the narrow walkway between the raised garden bed and the tall herbs growing against the old wooden fence. When I tire, or my arm becomes sore from casting, I walk in the house, instead of hiking two or three miles to the car parked under the trees above Mossy Creek, and a two-and-a-half-hour drive home. Sitting in a lonely room is often more soothing and mentally alive. It is easier to dream while I can, before Alzheimer steals the minutiae of my life.

> The young bike rider came down the long incline, her hair blowing away from her face, exposing a lovely smile. Then came the heavy struggle up the next hill, accompanied by a slow, methodical rhythm that required all the strength of her strong legs. Sweat beaded on her contorted face as she stood up to power-pump the bike. She reached the top, breathless and ready for the long glide ahead of her. Then she was gone.

I lost the little imaginative boy in me to greenhouses and it caused me to trade words for dirt. It took many years to weary me of dirt and I traded an outdoor life for one in a small, bright room.

Alzheimer's provided me an opportunity to give up dirt and search the rocky hillsides of memory for places where freshets remained to tell me who I was and where I have been. All around me I am greeted by my past, familiar places of memories from baby days to dying days, almost all in the same little community.

All the places I lived, the 14th Street of the forties and the 9th Street of the fifties, added up to angry days of standing apart from tradition in the Powhatan of the sixties. I walked in the wake of war and wasted talents. I inhabited schools named Walter Reed, Swanson and Washington-Lee for twelve years. The latter part of those years were marred by schoolboy anxiety and by frightening conflict over desegregating schools.

Years of silence coat the streets of my floundering memory. Trees sing to me as I walk through the remains of memory, while around me the world changes quickly before my hungry eyes. The sin of bulky high-rise buildings now shades a time of failing memory and nervous decline.

❧

THERE WAS A TIME, when the world was small, a boy looked up to his father with wonder and laughter. A father's very motion was filled with symbolism and fraught with magic. In that time, as now, fathers were not yet used to themselves. If they were honest, they kept trying to discover the person whose face stared back at them from the bathroom mirror.

I watched my father search for himself in many ways but his chief preoccupation was with his Italian roots and he sought them assiduously in the kitchen. It was in the kitchen he sought to link memory and aroma to cook special food *alla Nonna*.

Nonna is Italian for "granny." She was born Rosa Baresi in 1859 in Varmo, a village in what is now the Italian province of Friuli. There are grandmothers such as Rosa in every family. Our Nonna became for us who followed a giant, mythological figure and her culinary feats became legendary. My father placed her in his kitchen pantheon above everyone else.

Nonna was as close to Italy as my father came. Trying to understand the food she cooked was a way he understood himself. To my father, Italy was not just a place but a boot-shaped precipice on the map of his imagination. His father's eager and immediate acceptance of the new world he discovered in America began the next generation's search for itself in the myth and mystery of the past.

When the family ventured into the spiritual pathways of the kitchen, it was my father who led us. These special occasions when he cooked dinner found my mother, sister and me alive with anticipation, waiting anxiously all day, or even through several days of preparation, while he patiently cooked a tomato sauce for hours.

As I look back on these moments in the kitchen with my father, they are almost like a séance in which, by reenacting the remembered motions of his Nonna, she came alive. I knew, in my small world as a child, this cooking was less about food than about being. My father searched for something or somebody who was tied to Nonna's apron.

We all enjoyed my father's search for himself in the kitchen. It swept us along an aromatic current of ingredients as he experimented on the stove in an effort to duplicate the dishes he remembered from his childhood visits to Nonna's kitchen. I remember with laughter my father's sporadic episodes in the kitchen with the pots and pans and foreign aromas. It also brought throat-tightening sadness as he drifted in a sea of uncertain memories, the most dangerous way to explore the unknown.

> Playfulness has run away from me. I feel as empty as a piece of glass, and alone. No one can imagine what it is like to live in the Alzheimer's world where thoughts die before they cry.

Every day that summer the sun rose early and by noon temperatures nudged an unhealthy one hundred degrees. Water supplies dwindled and the county placed a ban on watering plants. These were serious days for my plants. All my stock plants from which new plants are grown were at risk of dying from lack of rain. I had never gone through such a thing before and I was scared.

With such high temperatures water evaporated quickly

from the ground. Fissures opened the dry earth. I began watering early in the morning and again in late afternoon. At greatest
risk were my boxwood. I bought young plants to grow for cuttings to root and they were only a few years old. These plants
were a centerpiece for my burgeoning greenhouse sales but now
I wondered if they could survive this hellish summer.

For three months there was no rain, only the high, hot sun.
My arms, legs and face were burned dark tan, visual marks of
the battle against unknown devils working to destroy my
dreams. In September the rains came and the drought lifted. I
lost few plants and my little emerging herb plant business was
saved.

I am on the brink of oblivion yet I find myself laughing because nobody sees inside where all the old truck
bodies are piled and rusting away.

My father desired Italian sheep cheese with texture and aroma.
It was necessary for his soul. Before long it was an obsession. It
was *pecorino formaggio* for which he went looking and it was
pecorino formaggio he could not find.

His determination finally led him to a little store on Lee
Highway in Arlington and he came home with a large smile.
He passed the cheese around to each of us so we could properly
appreciate his triumph. It was a little triangle with a creamy
center and a tan rind on the wide end. We thought it was a
smelly little piece of cheese wrapped in white paper. Up to then
I only recognized yellow cheese.

My father treated the little package of *pecorino formaggio* as if
it were a sliver of the True Cross and he secreted it in the altar of
his kitchen. Every Sunday, he reached into the cabinet next to
the sink and pulled out the little can into which he had put the
cheese. He brought the package into the light, and carefully
remove its cheesecloth wrapping. He laid it out on the cutting

board and pinched off a little piece, held it to the light and then quietly, as if receiving the Holy Sacrament itself, he deposited it on his tongue.

After a few months, the allure of the sacramental *pecorino formaggio* vanished and it was forgotten. The cheese sat in the can beside the sink "aging" until it could be used in the perfect culinary moment. One day I came into the kitchen to find my mother on her knees searching for something. There's an awful smell coming out of the drainpipe in the sink, she said to me by way of explanation and turned back to her task.

Finally, her hand landed on the cheese can. She placed it on the counter and gingerly opened the container and a foul smell permeated the room. The *pecorino formaggio,* kept as Nonna kept it, had expired and required a quick and proper burial.

Nobility may be the regal spine of failure, but when you stumble in search of yourself, there are surprising discoveries to be made.

> My mind used to be crowded with ideas. Now it is mostly empty except on unusual days like this one.

We knew basements. Our first was on the other end of a cement stairway. We wondered why there was a hole in the wall for the water to enter the basement. The hole in the wall was created to direct water into a drainpipe connected to the sewer. Unfortunately the rain often came with more force than the drain was designed for, and little boats sometimes bobbed on the basement floor.

When we moved to Ivy Street the basement was freshly washed and the old cinder blocks colored with white paint. We wondered why there were small, round holes in several areas of the room. We soon learned about water and old houses. A heavy storm pounded us and we looked in the basement at three inches of water standing on the concrete floor. It was then we learned why there were holes in the basement floor. It was a primitive way of removing water from the basement without a pump. We also learned the wooden stairway into the basement was installed before the concrete was poured. As the wood rotted, additional avenues of water haunted us.

Water was not the only problem with the basement of a too old house. In winter mice found ways into the basement. It appeared they found entry where the siding and the cinder block met. Most of the time the mice were well hidden. Once or twice our cats found a mouse or two and brought them upstairs to share the fun with us. I once watched a mouse climb the cinder block walls while our cats, much heavier, tried to climb after it.

My head used to be full of ideas and memories. Now hardly a moment of yesterday waves its flag at me. Upon my shoulder sits a vessel emptying itself of life.

My father loved fried cornmeal mush. He bought it at the Safeway in Westover right after the war. It came in little squares, clear packages through which you could see its golden skin shimmer. On Saturday morning, there was much joy when my father fried the square of firm cornmeal. While it was still hot from the griddle, he anointed it with real maple syrup or real butter. I don't remember whether it was the butter or the syrup, both of which had been in frustratingly short supply during the war, but I loved the song of that glorious combination of wealth and poverty. Fried cornmeal mush was simple, plain food but it was special in our house in the East because it was a link to both Iowa, where it was basic to survival, and to the myths of Varmo in Italy.

Along with the cornmeal mush went stories of Nonna and polenta. The cornmeal dish was common among the immigrant families from Friuli who immigrated to Des Moines, Iowa, where my father visited in his youth. Talking about polenta made Dad hungry for the memory of Nonna and her cooking.

Before many weekends had passed a big bag of yellow corn-meal appeared on the kitchen counter and it was announced that henceforth we would make our own polenta. There was no more cornmeal mush from the store.

Soon after the cornmeal mush pronouncement, my father stood before the stove like a priest celebrating Mass. He began the polenta ritual, unknown to any of us, by lighting the burner and placing a big pan of water on it. Once the water boiled, he began to add the cornmeal slowly, stirring at the same time. Cooking it took a long time, but soon it was ladled onto plates and we sat around the drop-leaf table watching the steam rise from the yellow mound on each plate.

During the war, we massaged plastic bags with a dot of yellow coloring gradually spreading through the colorless margarine. Then we dropped soft slices of it on the mounds of polenta and began to eat.

This polenta was quite different from the smooth cornmeal mush. It was gritty and had big lumps in it. There are times when misbegotten tradition must give way to modernism. Cornmeal mush was soon back in the refrigerator. Iowa triumphed over Friuli, at least for a while.

Even with its unkempt appearance, the garden's plants shine with brilliance. The silver lavender foliage floats above the underbrush of weeds like silver clouds.

The tomato sauces laboring through time, the lumpy polenta, the exotic spoiled cheeses, these were nothing compared to potato gnocchi, the crowning culinary achievement of the poverty-stricken Friuliani. Nonna's gnocchi were incomparable, according to my father, light as a feather with a depth of flavor complemented by a long-simmered tomato sauce.

One unforgettable Saturday, when the world was small, my father set about instructing me in the composition and cooking of these savory little dumplings. It was an unfamiliar dish I had never seen or eaten and which he had never attempted to cook. Dad dug into his memory deeply to remember the moves Nonna made. He boiled the potatoes first. He peeled them and mashed them in the mixer. He put the mashed potatoes in the center of a cutting board and added eggs, and flour. This was mixed by hand and kneaded carefully.

Finally, he stood back and let the dough stand with a cloth over it. In about an hour, he uncovered the dough and began taking little, sticky pieces from it which he rolled into balls and pressed against a cheese grater. He placed the gnocchi on a plate and soon the lumps of dough turned into soft, little shell-like objects with ridges.

While they sat on the plate, Dad got the large, deep spaghetti pot and filled it with water, to which he added the gnocchi. Then he lit the burner under it. We waited for the water to boil and the gnocchi to float to the surface.

The little potato dumplings refused to rise to the top of the boiling water. Something had gone wrong. He turned off the fire under the pot and poured out the water. There was a big sticky glob in the bottom of the pan; it was scraped into the trash. I learned much later the trick to make gnocchi rise is to put the uncooked potato balls into vigorously boiling water a few at a time.

I was happy food was around me when my world was small. It allowed me to learn that food was less important to sustain our bodies than it was to feed the secret places inside us where our true selves reside. When Dad made the attempts to recreate the part of himself he thought was hidden, I was not old enough to understand the symbolism of the food, or the necessity for the search.

For many people, history is a chronicle of past events put down in words and printed in books. For me, memory is more fleeting and personal and is found in the food, fragrances and gardens illuminating the windows to memory. This thing we call memory can be random and fitful but it has a special power of its own. It permits dead souls to animate the present and form rich undercurrents in still lives.

I watch stones float on water.

Remember the days of my dying. There were many. Monday, Tuesday, Wednesday, Thursday, Friday, Saturday and Sunday. Seven days a week, week after week.

Weeks walked into months of trembling and forgetting until there were no longer memories to remember.

Months stretched into years as my brain slowly wasted away until there was so little there was nothing to say and no way to say it. I counted more weeks until I was so weak there was little I could do but watch and wait in silence. Yet there was more horror to encounter.

In the darkness and confusion I was still and the mourners came to rescue the dead with words of yesterdays. They rattled memories while drinking beer until there was nothing more to be said. It was time for the next bonfire.

✼

As the car bumped slowly along the one-lane dirt road, a faded red pickup with rusting body came into view. It sat on the weed-choked berm. The driver's door hung open as if the truck had been abandoned hastily.

"There's Mario," said Jim Simon from the back seat of the car. I looked to the left of the pickup, toward the open field, in the direction Simon's arm pointed. A dark-haired, tanned man with a sheaf of papers in his left hand walked away from us through straight rows of basil plants. He was the man in a hurry to get out of the pickup.

Laura Clavio, a journalist and a friend, was driving the car, and she eased it off the road and stopped behind the pickup. I had come halfway across the U.S. for Simon to show me the future of basil and it was now in front of me in a lonely, mud-dark, Indiana field.

Simon came to Purdue University in West Lafayette, Indiana, as a vegetable crops specialist with a solid research background and a Ph.D., but he could not submerge his interest in herbs and alternative food crops.

Simon waded into the muddy field without hesitation, eager to show us the promise of his research. Each short row of plants in the field was marked with a numbered wooden stake. The sheaf of papers Morales carried contained information about the source of the seed that produced each row of plants. Bright, little plastic flags on stiff wire stanchions marked plants within rows or stood at the end of other rows. The flags designated plants showing promise for the scientists. Seed was collected from them for next year's crop.

This selection process began the first year and is performed each year as the plants' characteristics are evaluated. In this time-consuming way, breeders create from genetic diversity uniformity in plants produced from seed. There were many things for Simon and Morales to evaluate about each plant in every row; among them were the stature of the plant, leaf color and size, vigor and survivability, flowering characteristics, uniformity of the row and aromatic components. The two scientists visited the plants so often they knew the intimate details of each plant but there remained a palpable air of insecurity about their own evaluations.

Simon looked pleased and turned around. "Anybody have second thoughts?" he asked. Our host was anxious to leave this field of dreams to see some of his finished projects. He had good reason to show off. It contained a remarkable selection of lemon basils, particularly the richly scented one he named for his daughter, Dani.

It was soon time for me to return to Indianapolis for the plane ride home, and with the four of us in the front seat of the red pickup we raced back through the West Lafayette evening traffic jam caused by the emptying of the university. Back at the horticulture building Simon and I hopped into his little red car and drove out through the traffic to the interstate.

When I left Indiana in the late sixties after a short stint as a small town newspaper reporter, I never dreamed of a return to the state or thought of it as Basil Country, but here I was on this late summer evening in the Indianapolis International Airport with just such a thought in my head.

I watched my bag roll out of the X-ray machine and I grabbed it and looked up. On the other side of the security area stood the man who worked so hard to create this new image of Indiana and of herbs. Simon stood there waving good-bye to me with his right hand, a tired smile on his stubbled face. His left hand held his dinner, a huge slice of cheese pizza he had purchased to eat on the car ride back to West Lafayette, where his office, his lab, his basil fields and the future awaited him.

I look at the image reflected in the bathroom mirror. Head to chest, it looks like me, bashfully skinny. I look carefully, inspecting the face, eyes and chest for some outward sign of the disease leading me into the forever darkness. I do not understand the shape of the foreigner in my mind eating memory away, leaving me with language often unintelligible and full of gaps slow to fill.

When enough years had passed to call me man, but not enough to make me adult, I got a job in a tailor shop. It was a perfect place for such a time in a young man's life. There was opportunity to discover much about humanity, but I passed up the big lessons of life and stayed only long enough to discover everything I needed to know about the diversity of human taste.

The idea for the job was to legitimize the idea of leaving home, a difficult emotional predicament for parents as well as children. Leaving home is as highly desirable as it is often difficult. The purpose is always the same, although sometimes masked: to be on your own with a chance to create yourself whole, a state of being with great appeal for teenagers and poets.

I had two regular chores at the shop. I pressed pants, and I packed boxes with altered military uniforms to be sent around the country to their owners. This was done in a back room inhabited by two seamstresses and two tailors. The seamstresses were permanent fixtures, one a long, youthful African-American, the other a compressed white-haired woman with a heavy Yiddish accent. The tailors were rotated every few months by the company, brought up from Mexico. The banter carried on among the four of them was conducted in a language invented by their ethnicity, and it brought much laughter and confusion to the room.

I had some familiarity with packing boxes, but I had to learn how to use a big steam press, a piece of equipment as foreign as Mars to me. I learned to coordinate the pressure of the large top of the machine with the release of the steam from a foot pedal. Producing a straight crease in trousers was a long time coming. The job I liked least was pressing pants that desperately needed a good cleaning.

The two seamstresses, who also complained about working on unclean garments, found another use for the press, creating a sweet, pungent aroma to mask the sour aroma of tired trousers. As lunch approached, they placed foil-wrapped parcels from home on top of the press. The aroma of their lunches warming on the press turned a boring hour into an anticipatory delight, shared by everybody in the store, including customers.

The Mexican tailors had their own ritual, although it was mostly silent. They pulled out glass jars of hot green peppers and carried them to a large cutting table behind the seamstress sewing machines. They sat cross-legged on the table and opened the jars to the accompaniment of a sharp whoosh of air. They threw chilies into their mouths and chewed with great passion. Within five to ten minutes the jars were empty.

I thought I learned all there was to know about the wonderful variety of lunch in this little store. I had not come to know Jimmy well enough. Jimmy owned the dry cleaner down the street and he did a lot of work for the tailor shop. His shop gathered clothes in the morning for collection by a cleaning firm, returned in late afternoon for pickup. This left Jimmy with a lot of time on his hands during the day, and he liked to come to the tailor shop to talk. Jimmy was from Lebanon, with a pretty heavy accent, and he fit into the patois of the back room.

One day he asked me to have lunch with him. I was in Jimmy's shop many times to drop off uniforms to be cleaned after alterations were made, but I had never seen what was behind the front counter. For lunch, Jimmy took me behind the counter and beyond the racks of the clothes to the place in the store where he lived. He slept in a little cubicle on the left behind a drape. Opposite his sleeping quarters was a similar stall with a hot plate.

Jimmy motioned to me to have a seat on his bed while he fired up the hot plate. When it glowed, he pulled out a stained old skillet and set it on the hot plate. While it heated, he added a generous amount of olive oil. He put the olive oil can down and plunged his hands into a grocery bag out of which he pulled a white cauliflower. He cleaned it quickly and cut it in half with a single swat of a cleaver. He dropped the cauliflower pieces in the skillet where they sizzled and spat for a while.

When they were soft, he forked them onto slices of white bread and sifted some grated cheese on them. I was about to laugh in bewilderment when he looked at me and with a smile he said, Let's eat.

He wasn't kidding. His mouth opened wide and his teeth severed a piece of his cauliflower sandwich. I took a hesitant first bite and discovered something beautiful. The heat and the olive oil enriched the simple, outcast cauliflower, making it a vegetable of savory beauty.

It was in this way that a job turned into more than an apprenticeship. It became an introduction to a new life.

I search for the truth. Sometimes I feel it in my grasp, but it is an elusive concept. Truth carries its opposite. Time may change Truth's song, but the idea lives on. Truth is probably a concept we don't need to live our lives. Fantasy is sometimes more nourishing.

Art is not there to make the world a better place.
— Norman Rosenthal, Exhibitions Secretary,
British Royal Academy

❧

I found myself admiring the huge mound of chervil in the cold frame as the early morning sun warmed the late March earth. I leaned against a small spade and the sun beckoned me into a spring mood. Warm rays slanted through the cold frame's plastic covering and exploded in a haze over the plants. There was a mystical air to the scene.

There is nothing like the chervil of the early spring, a plant remarkably nourished by the hard, cold winter, but it is gone to seed so soon. It is a good thing to see it plump and full after a mild winter, rather than puny and milked of vitality by the sun and heat of summer. I cut a handful of chervil and sniffed its greenness and the hint of anise in the leaves and put it in the plastic bag I carried into the garden on such forays.

> And I hope that the Sixth Avenue El will remain
> what it always has been—a thing of horror and of
> beauty, so that forlorn poets staggering out of cozy
> restaurants will be reminded of simple things and
> long to communicate with the world.

> —HENRY MILLER, LETTER TO WILL SLOTNIKOFF,
> IN *The First Time I Live,* BY WILL SLOTNIKOFF

ALTHOUGH I HAVE never regarded myself as The Hermit of Ivy Street, it wasn't until early last winter that I realized how insular I was.

My self-awakening began with a drive beyond the beltway. I was surprised at the clogged roads. I envisioned a world nearly unpopulated, empty except for the open farmland and the occasional woodlot. It was more than unfamiliar; it was another world of which I knew less than a little.

This other world reminded me in many ways of my childhood. In those days, before Arlington was urbanized, men had rough hands and spoke softly and politely to children and anybody's mom could tell you how to behave without fear of contradiction. It was a place where cows munched grass on the hilly ground not far from Seven Corners, and swampy fields near the old Washington & Old Dominion railroad tracks held pulsing life in tiny frogs we called spring peepers.

My current insularity prevented me from knowing whether the verities of my childhood were present in the lives of those who lived in the houses by which I drove. It was the openness, the large sky and the incompleteness everywhere that recalled those unfinished, striving places I remembered from half a century ago.

Loudoun County recommended itself to me. It was my past

with a new frontier. Joyce and I actually looked at a greenhouse along Route 50 about twenty years ago and thought about purchasing it and the brick house behind it before we decided to stay put.

Soon after my sojourn in the country, Francesco and I began hanging around with a real estate agent named Bill Hunt. He took us to remote areas to look at land and buildings. After several weeks, we pulled up in front of a tumbledown place.

Francesco and I fell in love with the barn on this place of high grass, rabbits, deer, groundhogs and an assortment of biting insects. It was an exquisite brick edifice of three stories, a bit tattered now over sixty years after its construction. Maybe we should have taken my daughter-in-law Tammy's advice. "Why do you want an old, rundown place like that?" she asked pointedly after the home inspector left. Her question was practical and realistic. Of course, she was right to question our sanity. On the other hand, we had seen something hidden beneath the tall grass, mud and dilapidated buildings. We saw the germ of a dream, perhaps the same impulse pushing me years ago.

From the beginning, we called the new place "The Farm," but as a description it was a bit off the mark. It has only five acres, a far cry from the acreage required in the old days to pasture cows or produce corn, beans and alfalfa. It was not the space, its grass or its past urging us to think of it as a farm. It was the large, three-story brick and stone barn that dominates the space that called forth the word "farm" to describe it.

We like to pretend the farm is out in the country, but it is only a thirty-minute drive from Arlington. The land looks wild and free as long as you face the woods or peek at the high grass meadow across the street where weary farm buildings sit in a forlorn snit. You can also look out on the front lawn and find four or five deer eating grass. It is the kind of place where city slickers take seriously a failing septic field and are able to survive on the rumor that a real sewer line is on its way.

Francesco and Tammy took up residence in one of the two houses on the farm, after spending two months remodeling the interior of the little stone house. They turned it into a place of smiles and warmth. During summer, we worked hard to begin the transformation dictated by our dream. Among the first things we did was to remove an old, sagging shed improbably sited on the front lawn. On the same day, earthmoving machines also removed the little forest growing through a concrete pad where a chicken house once stood.

Greenhouses were ordered, a lawn tractor purchased and, most important, wonderful acquaintances were made among our new neighbors. By September's end, an herb farm in embryo could be seen, but there were few herbs in the ground to herald it.

In *Acres and Pains,* a book describing his adventures as a farm owner, S. J. Perelman wrote that "to lock horns with Nature, the only equipment you really need is the constitution of Paul Bunyan and the basic training of a commando." In time, I hope to discover whether the humorist was a sage or just a wisecracker.

I now see love and laughter as emotions close to tears.

I can feel the memories just beyond the depth I can reach, under the surface of awakening. It is a place uninhabited by words, full of the refuse of poets who never showed themselves. In my trance, words appear in a rapid spill, a magical creek bobbing with laughter and song. Small miracles still take place in my brain.

Memory now brings tears more often than laughter.

My cat Sabina helps me through this scruffy ordeal with Alzheimer's with dripping sentimentality and trembling, wet fear. She is a familiar part of my life and offers total attention.

The strong purring sound she makes when I stroke her furry back helps relieve my anxiety. In her silent way, she understands the peculiarities of humanity, and knows fear in an instinctual way humans have lost.

Guttural sounds choke my mouth, trembling screams without fathers, lost animal cries of rage.

I have gardened since I was five years old, more than fifty years, and I don't understand life without a spade in my hand and soft, rich soil in which to grow things. Gardening is so commonplace in my life I take the earth and dirty knees and summer-fresh vegetables for granted. This familiarity may be why it took me so long to realize the power gardening has over our common humanity.

I discovered the deeper meanings of the garden and the earth through the flinty evil of commerce. It did not happen in a flash of profit, but through the slow accumulation of experience, particularly encounters with dirt and flesh. I waited several years before I expressed it in the tilth of language. I noticed an involuntary willingness to make my discovery public in 1985, the year I marked the tenth anniversary of my garden business.

I sat down at my typewriter to prepare the spring catalog and the words and emotions I felt gushed down the page. What started as juju advertising copy became an eyeball-to-eyeball chat with the most important people in my life at the time—my customers who came every spring to buy herb and vegetable transplants for their gardens. These strangers with an interest in dirt and herbs gave me a sense of belonging for the first time in my life and a lot of my anger and alienation slipped away as my contact with them continued.

I got a glimmer something unusual was afoot when I received presents from these strangers. They were not big gifts, just homemade stuff: bottles of herb vinegar, seed packets of unusual European plants, a jar of honey, raspberry liquor, cookies, cheeses, bags of herb-flavored popcorn, a favorite recipe or a bottle of coriander chutney. I have worked at a number of jobs—store clerk, adult education teacher, picture framer, journalist, editor and truck driver—but I never received such an outpouring of love and respect. Customer is too crass a word to describe the folks who buy my plants.

In lonely times of winter, when the hours are long and unrelieved and nature is unyielding, I think of the thousands of people who have been drawn to my garden, people from my immediate neighborhood and throughout Virginia, as well as those from Annapolis, Bowie, Adelphi, Rockville, West Virginia, North Carolina, Delaware, Connecticut, Ohio, North Carolina and all the faraway places I can't remember. The memory of their smiles and enthusiasm sustains and nurtures me.

Money is a crass value placed on a business like mine. The riches are in the people I have been privileged to meet and the warm friendships that developed, even the seasonal ones. It is sad when a customer calls to tell me a spouse or a friend died or is sick. It is an honor to be invited to their weddings, baptisms and funerals and to be let in on their secrets. They have taught me much over the years, and this book is as much their work as it is mine. They taught me to look at the world differently.

> René Magritte was often moved by brief flashes of illumination. One day he saw his wife eating a chocolate bird, and immediately produced an image of a young woman eating a live bird, with its blood flowing over her hands. On another occasion a glimpse of the lathe-turned feet of a table inspired him to paint the huge wood-turnings of the landscape in *Annunciation*.
>
> —SARANE ALEXANDRIAN, *Surrealist Art*

As I walk along the sidewalk, the early morning promenade of automobiles has begun. One after another they hurtle down the road like race drivers on an empty holiday. Some drivers eat breakfast as they hurry along to work. The air vibrates with the energy of the gasoline combustion engine. In this leafy green community a sniff away, I manicure the landscape with words.

Many days I hover gently between awareness and emptiness.

I looked around the garden. Winter winds blow leaves and trash everywhere. I have to begin spring cleaning soon. The best part of the early season is pruning the lavenders, a task I have ritualized. Each spring I prune these hardy plants by removing one-third to one-half of the length of each stem. It is time-consuming work, but necessary. The pruning provides me an opportunity to shape the plant, but more important it encourages new branches, the source of sweet, new lavender flowers. Left unpruned, lavender becomes procumbent and highly susceptible to fungus diseases. On unpruned plants, the center turns woody and twisted, laying the plant open to the deadly ravages of winter. There is so much to do in the spring it can leave a gardener breathless.

My memories reside in a glass repository. One day I pulled the glass out of its hiding place and turned it upside down. The water poured out, splashing away in rivulets, dispersing my memories and leaving me wandering without a map. I watch with sorrow as the liquid in the glass disappears.

I moved down the garden path, flourishing a small spade like a walking stick. The spade was unusual and is one of my favorites, rather long and narrow with a dished blade and a yellowish wooden handle smoothed by use.

I stopped in a shady spot under a tree littered with leaves. I brushed away the debris. There were little green shoots rising from a tangle of roots that ran riot over the soft, dark ground. It was time to divide the sweet woodruff.

I thrust the spade into the earth to the right of a clump of woodruff and then jabbed it into the ground on the left, then forward and back. I lifted the little square of earth with the roots running though it. I massaged it with my right hand until the dirt crumbled away and I saw the runners with their little green shoots. The wispy hair of the roots hung in clumps.

With a pair of scissors from my pocket, I cut the runners so each piece had a clump of roots and some new growth. I took these sweet woodruff divisions around to the other side of the tree, loosened the ground a little with the spade. I picked up the small root divisions and shoved them into the earth, spacing them about six inches apart.

I went to the basement for the watering can, brought it back filled to the brim, and poured the water on the transplants. It was cool enough here and the sun did not hit the new divisions. I got away with planting them directly in the ground, something I would not dare do later in the year. In summer's heat it is necessary to pot the young plants first and let the divisions become well rooted and adjusted to their new life before transplanting them.

I hoisted the spade over my shoulder with the empty watering can swinging from it and happily headed for the sorrel, where I intended to perform the same horticultural surgery. On a spring day like this, the senses tingle with anticipation and the earth becomes a huge clock marking time in slow movements, preparing seasonal life and regeneration.

*   *   *

Human beings make a strange fauna and flora.
From a distance they appear negligible; close up
they are apt to appear ugly and malicious. More
than anything they need to be surrounded with
sufficient space even more than time.

—Henry Miller, *Tropic of Cancer*

～

In my family, the idea of landscaping was held in contempt, but
vegetable and herb gardens were sacred. This all came about
over the years as we turned practicality into a stern morality to
guide us.

I learned this code long before I picked up a shovel of my
own. It was taught by my father's example and the story he told
of my grandfather's encounter with his father many years before
my birth.

My great-grandfather was named Domenico when he was
born June 3, 1850, the second of five children born to Antonio
and Rosa Di Biassio in the village of Romans-di-Varmo in the
province of Udine in a region the Italians call Friuli. Peasants
have struggled for centuries against weather and earth in this
part of Italy and they stayed alive by growing food in gardens,
and by hunting. In my great-grandfather's time, the women of
Romans worked in a factory, spinning thread from the cocoons
of worms into silk.

None of these enterprises created the life Domenico or his
younger brother, Francesco, wanted, and they came to the fertile
soils of America to find another life. Even in this eager new land,
the ways of thinking in Romans-di-Varmo marked them forever.

The religion of the men of Friuli was nominally Roman
Catholic, but their true faith was practical and was based on

raising food. Domenico and Francesco spent much of their lives in Italian and American gardens. They were priests of its peasant ritual.

Those who came after and were formed by the great abundance of Iowa and of the United States may never fully understand the depth to which this peasant religion of the garden penetrated the core of the Friuliani. My grandfather, who lived only eight years under this rite, was influenced little by it, and his father, Domenico, noticed this.

Great-grandfather Domenico visited his son soon after grandpa moved into a new house in Colfax, Iowa. In Iowa, the houses have extremely wide bands of grass between the street and the public sidewalks. We call these grass bands parkings for some reason, although nobody thinks of spoiling the beautiful grass by parking anything on it. In Iowa, the green swatch of parking is the rehearsal for the lawn.

Domenico lived in Des Moines, a short train ride from Colfax, and while my grandfather was called Harry by everyone in America, his father was stubborn and always called him Enrico, the name he gave him in Italy. Great-grandpa was unyielding in other ways, too. The old man walked over this wide, green parking and across the grassy lawn and grew angrier with every step. He burst into his son's new house spluttering in disbelief. "Enrico," he said, accusingly, "how can you waste so much land in unproductive grass when it ought to produce food? You have committed a grave sin."

> The fear of falling is the source of many a folly. It is a disaster. I suppose the wisest thing is not to live it over again, meditate upon it and be edified. It is thus that man distinguishes himself from the ape and rises from discovery to discovery, ever higher, towards the light.
>
> —Samuel Beckett, *Malone Dies*

The narrow road is smooth with woods on both sides. The car speeds along unpaved lanes covered with chunks of stone while I am full of memories from places I have never encountered.

Domenico was not the only Friuliano imbued with this moral outlook on the importance of gardens and fresh food. My grandmother, Lottie DeBaggio, sent me a newspaper clipping years ago which appeared in the *Des Moines Register* during the Great Depression. It shows a man identified as Frank DeBiaggio, my great-grandfather Domenico's brother, whom our family called Checco. He is wearing bib overalls, and a dark wool cap with a bill slanted to the right side of his head; earflaps are tied across his crown.

He is a grizzled old man and he does not hide his nearly eight decades of life on earth, but he has mischievous eyes and a firm, kind mouth. His cheeks are puffed up as if a smile is about to explode across his face. In his right hand, he holds a trowel. A watering can is beside him. You can almost smell the earth and manure even after all these years inside a photograph reproduced in a newspaper.

In the few lines the reporter wrote under the photograph, Checco extols the tomato plants in his greenhouse and foresees the delight they will bring during the warm summer when the fruits ripen in the garden. The caption goes on to say: "DeBiaggio plants only things to eat, because, he says, you can only smell flowers; they have no practical use." This is an idea from that same catechism taught by the Friuliani priests of the garden and it is not surprising that the brothers, Domenico and Francesco, shared it, too.

Two men pass each other silently on an empty sidewalk. As they hurry in opposite directions, rain begins to fall.

*   *   *

It did not take long before I realized the paucity of herb varieties in the U.S. I saw a place for my new business in what I sensed was a coming boom in gardening. Vegetables and herbs were the combination I chose to tease the palates of people my age. The established companies sold the same vegetable varieties every year, with few new varieties. It was a time when the old guard threw off a past of lush-flavored antique varieties, with their heavy burden of disease, but were not yet ready to create new varieties. Before long a flood of new vegetables inundated home gardeners.

I forsook the U.S. palate and sought European seeds. My approach was straightforward. I wrote letters to the embassies in Washington, D.C., asking for names of companies specializing in herb and vegetable varieties. I sent out about a dozen letters and within a few weeks I had catalogs from French and Italian companies. A French company offered leek seeds and I bought them. The seeds germinated and within a month or two I had seedling flats for sale.

From an Italian firm outside Salerno many items were ordered from a large, colorful catalog. The first items in the catalog were lists of American melons, from Charleston Grey to Sugar Baby, three pages of them. I wondered if America had overrun southern Italy. I paged ahead quickly and found the remainder of the catalog full of Italian goodies. I was overwhelmed with the five different basils. I expected them, but not the *cardonetto,* the *groccolo,* the *carciofo,* the *cardo.* The Finocchio (nine varieties) overwhelmed me. The fourteen varieties of Rapa were unbelievable. I puzzled over the thirty different *cicoria.*

Mennella offered seeds in packets and in sacks. I ordered large sacks of the basils, *Genovese grande violetto, Napoletano verde, Nano compatto* and *Piccolo verde fino,* as well as packets to sell. Among the vegetables I ordered tomatoes: Cuor di Bue, San Marzano Lampadina Extra, Nano a Grappoli and Marzano. I went crazy ordering items from the catalog. It was like coming home starved, and I dug in.

Every year I ordered from Mennella in the complex way it had to be done, with money sent in advance and a long wait, sometimes months. I found the lead time was half a year but it was worth it. Nobody had these super varieties. After fifteen years, I got a letter from Italy. Mennella had closed and returned the money for my last order. I cried bewildered tears. My tears were wasted. Many companies had by then tapped into European seeds.

> Perhaps I am doomed to retrace my steps under the illusion that I am exploring, doomed to try and learn what I should simply recognize, learning a mere faction of what I have forgotten.
>
> —André Breton, *Nadja*

September 18, 1992

Dear Linda,

I'm sorry you've had such a number of emotional shocks this summer. I know such things can make it difficult to concentrate on anything for long. You are right about the valuable role books play in the healing process. I think gardening acts on the mental pressure points in much the same slow way.

> I will have to revisit all the places I've been miserable in, just to see if I can be happy in them after all.
>
> —Paul West, *The Rat Man of Paris*

It happened one day as the world teetered between summer and fall. No leaves turned from green to yellow or orange or brown.

No geese honked into view and appeared silhouetted against the gray sky in a wobbly, slow-moving V. It was a day when the earth remained warm from the sun of summer and the air was cool and heavy with moisture and messages.

As I stood with a hose in my hand watering lavenders, a familiar scent came to me. It was not a sweet herbal aroma, nor a scent from the donut shop down the street. It was a scent bringing the past and all its memories with a rush. I don't know how to explain such a scent without sounding foolish or mystical. I can say this much: it was a complex perfume of Prince Albert pipe tobacco, hard work, old clothes and the kitchen aromas of frying meat, steam rising from boiling vegetables, gravy and baking pies.

The scent that reached my nose was the distinct, remembered aroma of my grandfather, born of restaurant kitchens, his pipe and the Midwest farming town of Eldora, Iowa, where he lived. It was as if he were next to me, looking over my shoulder, and I turned involuntarily first to my left and then to my right, half expecting him to be there. There was no one; my grandfather has been dead for years.

Grandpa's aroma was in the air around this spot in the garden all morning and I walked around it and through it. The scent was the same each time, and it brought back a flood of memories.

My grandfather spent more than half a century in front of a hot stove in a series of restaurants he owned in small-town Iowa. That was long enough for him to be able to tell if food was seasoned properly by sniffing the steam that rose from the pan. I remember grandpa in his kitchen with no romanticism because I retain a memory of his battered legs, bandaged and plastered so he could stand another day with the varicose veins his restaurants gave him.

It is easy to sense the amazing poetry, energy and imagination that goes into the preparation of fine food. It is the part inside me that grandpa touched and I remember most vigorously. It was the odor of the hard work of cooking and the chaos in which anonymous cooks work. Grandpa always meant much to me because of my memory of him and the stories my father recounted of him. It is not often that we glimpse a father, a mother or grandparents in this way and it is a sight to hold and keep.

For most children, their parents' lives exist in remote shadows. Grandparents are often even more mysterious and their lives more remote.

The mystery of an earlier life inhabits a large space between parents and their children. When I was barely a teenager my father took my mother and my sister and me to Italy. It is clear to me my father went there to search for something of his own father that was missing.

The visit to the ancestral home in Romans-di-Varmo was ritualistic: the examination of the birth records in the old church, the search for my grandfather's birthplace. As a teenager, I was bewildered by all the women with deeply creased faces, dressed in black, who stared at us as we passed. The guttural language spoken by the Ladin-speaking Friuliani of this part of rural Italy in the province of Udine was something of a mystery even to our Venetian driver.

Romans-di-Varmo that day was little changed from the day my grandfather was born, December 24, 1883. This foreign place was a great mystery inside my father all his life. So I studied the sun and the way it looked in this village in Italy. I sought a clue to the child my grandfather had been here. My father went into the house he was told was my grandfather's birthplace. My mother, sister and I had to stay outside.

Denied this intimate bit of sightseeing, I inspected the dirt in the street to help me understand my grandfather. I was unaccustomed to this method of assaying the geology of the human soul and I learned little.

*   *   *

As I walk along the sidewalk on my daily stroll, two young women in Saturday pants go into the fortune-teller's house. It is a bright winter Saturday afternoon. There is a secret world everywhere I walk.

I don't know how long it has been this way, but during the nearly thirty years I have lived on Ivy Street there was only one occasion when residents battled each other seriously in court. I know the story because I lived between the two combatants and got sucked into their dispute.

When we moved into the house on Ivy Street, we knew someone lived in the house next to us, but they were so quiet we heard almost nothing from their side of the fence. As time passed, changes occurred. The largest was the greenhouses sprouting everywhere. They said nothing when I began to sell plants a few feet from their driveway.

It was soon evident a parking area was needed; the street was so narrow it was signed No Parking all around us. I expanded the small grassy area in front of the house, trading greenery for loads of pea gravel. It created a place large enough to park four cars in a pinch but it left no space for grass. Many customers parked under No Parking signs instead of parking on 10th Street where there was parking a few steps away.

Everything went well until the Navy officer who owned the house next to us put it up for sale instead of for rent. It sold quickly at a price high enough to be a surprise. The couple who bought it had no children but they soon adopted two.

About the same time, a rental house opposite us was refurbished. Everything was thrown out, floors were improved to a sparkle, and the son of the owner moved in. Hampton, we discovered early, was a good ol' boy in the best sense of the word. He was helpful when needed and he liked loud music, as did many people of his young age. His roommate was a young black man who floated away after a year. Hampton didn't like living alone and bought a puppy, a cute, little, active Rottweiler. If the loud music wasn't surly enough the dog's image exuded fear.

Before long I saw my next-door neighbor standing in front of Hampton's house. He was screaming for him to lower the volume. Then he knocked on the door. Two angry men greeted each other with disrespect. This went off and on for months and the decibels escalated. One day my next-door neighbor told me Hampton flipped his middle finger in a manner of disrespect to the neighbor as she drove their car past him, an act he denied. The neighbor went to court and brought charges against Hampton. All the corks popped and I was dragged into it as a witness.

There was a long wait before we went into the courtroom in Arlington. My next-door neighbor and Hampton both had attorneys representing them. The courtroom was small but it was plenty large enough for the three of us and the two lawyers. Both sides were questioned. After my testimony, the judge told Hampton and my neighbor to keep away from each other if they couldn't get along together.

With the problem with Hampton temporally shelved, my next-door neighbor focused on me. Their problems with me, or more exactly with my plant customers, were complex. Customers were parking in front of their house when my four-place parking lot was filled. Once or twice a thoughtless customer actually parked in their driveway, blocking them from egress. This job was for the woman of the house next door. She came knocking on our door late one night. She wanted us to do something about the parking congestion my little business created. She suggested better signs. We told her we would make larger signs and try to encourage our customers to be more considerate.

Joyce went to work, creating large, bright signs someone driving in a car could easily see. The signs were clear about parking. Several signs were ready within a few days and I installed them along the street, from my house to the main road. One was placed on the power line post separating our properties.

The next night there was a late knock on the door. It was our next-door neighbor. She was angry and nervous. She labeled our new large, bright signs unworthy. She wanted them taken down and replaced with signs of her design, dark things without eye appeal or information, and small. We put up several of these paper signs and let them blow away in time. It was not long before a For Sale sign appeared next door.

My grandmother, Lottie DeBaggio, sometime after the trip to Romans-di-Varmo, sent me a thin blue folder containing what she called the Family Tree. Within its pages are genealogical lists, and I turn to it when I want to enter the old world. I run my fingers down the names of family members going back to 1625 and try to imagine them: Mattia, Maria, Domenica, Giaccoma, Zuanna, Valentino, Maddalena, Antonio, Domenico, Pasqua, Sebastiano, Giovanni, Gucia, Cattarina, Giuseppi, Durando, Francesco, Rosa, Enrico and Anna. The names themselves call up emotions buried in the mists of time, but these feelings have all the permanence of steam escaping from an inactive volcano.

Those names on a family tree have been enough these last fifty years to place my grandfather in the world from which he came. But the world in which I saw my parents and my grandparents was one always circumscribed by the family; it was not the real world in which they spent most of their lives among genetic strangers.

I began to see my grandfather in a larger world when I read *The Fine Family of Nine,* a privately printed book compiled by my father's cousin, Peter Dawson. His book is a treasury of family stories, and he always cautioned me he took liberties to flesh out tales where facts were thin.

My grandfather earned a place in this book because his sister, Anna, became the second wife of Pete's father, Pietro Dapolonia. Anna was Pete's mother. Grandpa's special role in the marriage was bringing the two families together in America. It was his task, unwelcome and difficult, to convince his rigid father, Domenico, to permit the marriage of his seventeen-year-old sister to a widower nearly twice her age with two children to whom she was formerly their servant. Domenico forbade the marriage as unholy and immoral, and, of course, his wife, Rosa, would not cross her husband.

Grandpa was only a year and a half older than his sister, and he openly disagreed with his stern, stubborn father. When his father refused to sanction Anna's marriage, he gave away the bride at the wedding ceremony that his parents refused to attend. This act of disobedience and revolt against his father's moral code was unusual and important for me to know.

❋

I GOT TO the place during my walk that is within shouting distance of home. There was a crowd forming near the Episcopal church on the corner, opposite the newest construction site. From under the women's coats, I saw the long, blue taffeta dresses of the maids of honor. Behind them, men strode into the church in their black suits and glinting black shoes.

A single gull circles high in a sky split with aeronautic explosions. Contrasting streaks of contrail push away memories of fleeting childhood moments. The dark shivers with whispers and pink clouds.

During the day my blood runs red and thin, like a dream meandering through my body without a trace of a scream from the back of my throat. At night my blood sparkles inside my shut eyes as I try to sleep. I see flowers and folds of color, mostly the oceans of red but also tumbling falls of blues and hints of green moving at a fast pace.

Sometimes bright white lights blind me as if a speeding car headed toward me. At other times I see a river of red blood roll by in front of me, a stream out of its banks sweeping away everything in its path. It is on nights like this I sometimes awaken shaking with fear, honking from the back of my throat with a wild Alzheimer's scream.

> Can it be that this desperate pursuit comes to an end here? Pursuit of what I do not know, but pursuit in order to set working all the artifices of intellectual seduction.
>
> — ANDRÉ BRETON, *Nadja*

JANUARY 14, 1994

Dear Linda,

Over the last several years, I've had time to think about the structure of a sentence and to see how sentences make paragraphs, and how all this contributes to a writer's style, and the meaning of the words he chooses. It is true that you and Mr. Hemingway started me to think about all this, and I spent 1993 looking inside myself to see what was there. I found something although I denied it was there earlier. It is up to me to see where this all leads, but I like knowing it is there even if it leads nowhere.

*   *   *

One of the many curious and delightful things about our country is the ease with which our good people move from one religion to another, or from no particular religion at all to any religion that happens to come along, without experiencing any particular loss or gain, and go right on being innocent anyhow.

— WILLIAM SAROYAN, *My Name Is Aram*

The angel lay in the little thicket. It had no need of love; there was nothing anywhere in the world could startle it—we can lie here with the angel if we like; it couldn't have hurt much when they slit its throat.

— KENNETH PATCHEN,
The Journal of Albion Moon Light

I envy (in a manner of speaking) any man who has the time to prepare something like a book and who, having reached the end, finds the means to be interested in its fate or in the fate which, after all, it creates for him. If only he would let me believe that on the way at least one true occasion to give it up presented itself! He would have disregarded the chance, and we might hope he would do us the honor of saying why.

— ANDRÉ BRETON, *Nadja,*

AUGUST 4, 1994

Dear Linda,

As a junior high pupil, I was sent to the Don Pallini Dance School where I learned to smash the toes of wall flowers. I never learned to dance, although I got over my apprehension about holding females. Life taught me even when you dance alone, you can step on toes, but the digits most often smashed are your own.

Spring is a time of indulgence for gardeners, a chance to purchase dreams and to watch them grow like well-behaved children. When the doorbell rings and UPS has left a box of these dreams on the front porch, I come inside with a big smile under my mustache. One day the box may contain a dwarf thyme discovered by Cy Hyde of Well-Sweep Herb Farm in New Jersey; it's a little treasure with miniature leaves clustered together on wiry stems that grow about six inches high.

On another day a packing box will contain a new variegated creeping thyme that shows bright spots of gold through green like blinking lights. And yet another box, this one from Nichols Garden Nursery in Albany, Oregon, contains the latest conceit in lavender breeding from the West Coast. These are gems to enliven the chaos of a garden tended with haphazard enthusiasm.

Before new plants can be transplanted, they need to spend a week or two in my cold frame. This time in a protected but outdoor world gives the tender, new plants a chance to become acclimated, a process that toughens soft growth that would otherwise be damaged by wind, cold and harsh sun.

On the first cloudy day I head out early to fetch the plants and place them in the garden. I'm careful not to yank them from their pots; instead, I turn them upside down and squeeze the plastic until the plant falls gently into my other hand. Then I thrust my thumbs into the root system and spread them, a procedure that might make a timid gardener shudder. I am not timid in this regard because I know such violence will keep the roots from continuing to wrap around themselves, as they must in the pot, and help them spread into the earth quickly.

The ground has been long prepared for transplanting by adding plenty of humus and it is so soft I need no shovel, or even a dibble, to aid in the transplanting. Into the soil goes my left hand where it creates a small hole. The plant in the right hand goes into the hole and is twisted slightly to firm it. From the watering can comes a fine splash of liquid fertilizer.

You needn't be a gardener to feel the spring heal the earth and renew its life, but spring allows the gardener to participate in this renewal in a special, intimate way through sowing seeds and growing new plants. It also brings to the gardener special responsibilities of nurture and protection; gardeners grow things where Nature never intended them to be.

The narrow road is smooth and the car speeds along with no memories of bumps.

The modern world has made easier the successful nurturing of tender plants by gardeners. In recent years I've come to depend on spun-bonded polyester material (Reemay is one trade name for the stuff) when temperatures dip and to protect sorrel against the predation of leaf miners, which tunnel through the succulent foliage, leaving their wiggly, disfiguring, brown path through the big, sour, green leaves. The other day the temperatures felt warm enough to awaken the flying insects that lay the leaf miner eggs on the underside of sorrel (and spinach, beet, chard, and Good King Henry) leaves. I went to the basement, hunted up some used pieces of Reemay that were large enough to cover the sorrel, and threw it over the young, tender leaves. The light, woven fabric allows sun and water through it, but it easily blows away in the strong spring breezes if I don't mound dirt over its edges or place stones to hold it down.

Slugs are also a major problem in my spring garden when cool, damp weather and tender new growth beckon the slimy little herbivores to a garden feast. The real disaster is that they always pick on my herbs. Oh, how they entertain themselves in the dark on my basil seedlings! Why are they so attracted to sorrel, sage, peppers, marigolds and so many other garden plants? They will consume entire leaves in a single nightly feeding sometimes, leaving a seedling denuded. At other times, in a less gluttonous mood, they will eat only jagged pieces from around a leaf's edges or attack the middle.

Get 'em where they live has always been good advice. Slugs live under stones, along the sides of raised beds, beside fence posts—a thousand damp, dark places where they congregate in the slippery nether world. Unfortunately, that lonely jar lid of stale beer is overworked and not terribly effective against the hordes of ravenous slimy slug mouths. Copper flashing works much better, a trick any old snail raiser knows. Whitney Cranshaw at Colorado State University tested a new product called Snail Barr, a thin copper foil six inches wide. He found slugs won't cross a copper barrier because electrical charges develop between the slime trail and the metal. A kind of passive electric fence for slugs. Who can condemn the modern world for such ingenuity?

Those early crops of dill, rucola and coriander bring such joy to me that it's a shame they are so short-lived, but frequent cutting of the foliage will often prevent the inevitable flower stalks from appearing and announcing the end of foliage production. I still rely on succession planting of these tender, green crops. I plant the seeds directly in the ground in short rows in mid-March and add more rows about every four weeks until the end of August. When plants start to flower, I yank them up and use the space for a fresh row of seed.

New life begins in the garden no differently than anywhere else. Youth possesses few qualifications except rapid growth, and the plant, no less than the child, needs constant attention and pruning to remain true to itself and to mature with grace and aplomb.

OCTOBER 11, 1994

Dear Linda,

I am sorry to hear your father-in-law died and your mother is so ill. Joyce and I both know the shudder, anger and sorrow of the loss of a loved one and we send our love and sympathy to you and your family.

It was twenty-five years before I could properly grieve for my parents. The grieving began a year ago when I stood before their tombstones in a cold little cemetery as dawn's bright edge crept over the horizon in Eldora, Iowa. The tears came and I began to realize what their loss meant to me. Twenty-five years is an unnaturally long time to hide sorrow. I felt ashamed for waiting so long to cry over their bodies, but at the same time, the tears seemed to renew my spirit. Grief deepened my emotional reservoirs and heightened my sensitivity to the world.

Watching my parents waste away slowly left a memory both terrible and frightening, but choking back the tears and refusing to grieve was worse because it left an important part of my life barren. Now I realize the importance of grief and it comes to me much easier, sometimes almost every day for short moments. It is this grief that allows memories of the departed to take up residence inside us and grow into new appendages. In times like these, tears have the power to reinvigorate the poetry and value of life.

I have described before how closing my eyes at night brought a series of still photographs. These mild hallucinations, and the bright white light that accompanies them, have puzzled me most of the year. Only recently did I realize what they were telling me.

At first I thought I was in an audience, perhaps in an art

gallery. The other night I looked carefully at the visages and discovered there was perspective I missed. I realized I was looking at ethereal snapshots from a place below them, perhaps on the ground. Was I lying on silent, still grass, resting on my elbows on a warm green day? Perhaps I fell off my bike or tripped on small gravel on the sidewalk. I decided I was looking back at the earth while the dust of my ashes dispersed in the universe. The pictures with their stiff formality were showing me a world after I died.

> The tragedy of this world is that no one is happy, whether stuck in a time of pain or of joy. The tragedy of this world is that everyone is alone. For a life in the past cannot be shared with the present. Each person who gets stuck in time gets stuck alone.
> — Alan Lightman, *Einstein's Dreams*

> The first of these statues was Grouloulou, made of pieces of newspaper smeared with glue and bunched around an armature. It was above all a glorification of newspaper. I had only recently used torn fragments of newspaper in several assemblages, notably in the poster from my show at Cercle Volney. Groulouou was therefore closely related to these works.

> The second was Gigoton, made of steel wool such as housewives use to clean their pots and pans. The third, Personage with Past Eyes, made use of fragments of burned automobiles that I found in the garage where I kept my car.
> — Peter Selz, with text by the artist,
> *The Work of Jean Dubuffet*

*   *   *

Rob, I may need a jolt or two of Lourdes water before I am through. I am against experimenting with bee stings on people with Alzheimer's. See you on the mountain soon. Rob Lively is a good friend but a Christian.

Recently I began to watch my cat Sabina. I crept into the living room and found her meditating. She was in a deep trance, eyes barely open, twitching slightly, and not in the world but not sleeping either. She seemed almost lifeless but when I moved quickly, I realized she was waiting quietly for me in both worlds, the one in shiny life and one sheltered underground.

Writing is a world of its own. First it hovers in the mind, coagulates into sentences, then paragraphs appear and, if you are patient, the words turn into a book. It is at this point I lose interest and send it out into the world where you find it and stick your nose into it, and judge me.

NOVEMBER 21, 1995

Dear Art,

Francesco returned to begin work with me in the nursery eight weeks ago and I thought that would give me more free time. Where does it all go? Digging a four-foot-deep trench to keep the neighbor's bamboo from attacking us has taken much more time and effort than we thought, but so has everything else. Nothing is on time this fall. Where does all the time go. Down some metaphysical drain I suppose. Even arising at four-thirty a.m. doesn't seem to help.

With my name on three books, you would not expect me to have symptoms of a neophyte, but I tremble every day. Now a New York editor paws through my new word baby and I have never felt so unself-confident. And why not? This is the editor who asked me whether Joyce and I slept in the same bed.

Cold white lights haunt my waking dreams. Where does this stabbing, watery light come from? Does it have special meaning for me?

Most people don't take time to think about death. When death shows its head, it is impossible to put aside thoughts about the shortness of life and how little is accomplished while we live out our meager time. With Alzheimer's there is plenty of time to ponder death, too much really. It makes me want to be run over by a fancy car. Anguished days of confusion and unreadable secrets puff up time and bring sudden yelps and rainbows behind my eyes where the tears live.

DECEMBER 4, 1995

Dear Kathleen,

My bluster hides a tender insecurity. At its heart is the desire to control and manipulate the world, a large order for any kid from Iowa. When editors tinker, they tell me I was right to feel insecure and threatened. I am a writer without formal training and I have to inflate myself artificially to begin tapping the keys that produce words and sentences. What little talent I have is vulnerable to attack by every pencil pusher with a green eyeshade.

Linda Ligon has always been at the top of my list as an editor; she can massage my ego and shape my sentences, and make me feel good about it most of the time. A great editor can divine the meaning behind a clumsy para-

graph and wrestle it into the light. You are a worthy suc-
cessor to Linda and your bedside manner is from the
same clinic.

Without memory, each night is the first night,
each morning is the first morning, each kiss and
touch are the first. . . . In order to know himself,
each person carries his own Book of Life, which is
filled with the history of his life. . . . Without his
Book of Life, a person is a snapshot, a two-
dimensional image, a ghost.

—ALAN LIGHTMAN, *Einstein's Dreams*

Silent airplanes with trembling lights drop through the
dark night sky, celestial lights with a utilitarian purpose.

My garden is my life and my livelihood, and it has marked me
with its curse and its promise. This is not Eden and it makes no
pretense to be like one of those estate gardens fancy magazines
show in full color. This garden of mine is a humble working
garden in the temperate zone along the Atlantic Coast of the
United States, not the worst place to garden and not the ideal
either.

It is winter now and outside the large greenhouse, filling my
backyard, the garden is a pitiful, frozen thing in the cold winter
light. For a garden from which its farmer obtains his income, it
is stunning in its modesty, not 25 feet wide and 150 feet long. It
is an unkempt stretch of beds raised above the ground by
unpainted two-by-eights topped with tufts of foliage, stems and
a lingering fragrance of herbs. Straight gravel paths run the garden's length in a rigid, tan geometry scaring nature with its discipline. This may be a place of struggling beauty in summer but
it is, like my life, all that I require.

A garden is a place to work, a place to dig into the earth and bring forth life. It is also a place to drop to your knees and nurture young life and watch it mature. Most of my garden, like all gardens, is a place to dream. In winter, I dream of the promise and peculiarity of spring. Once spring arrives, I begin to dream of summer's warm earth with its splendid growth, rich aromas and bountiful harvests. In fall, my annual dreams become middle-aged. I sense the coming of autumn and savor the memories of bright springs with tender, young green shoots poking through bare, dark soil. In busy fall I fill paper bags with spent herb flowers to supply the garden with seeds full of still life. Every garden is a hidden Eden with a clock, a remarkable crucible to measure reality and its reflection, but which can warp the most finely etched memory.

It's hardly surprising to find the substance of poetry in gardens and I find myself hugging mystical thoughts for warmth on a cold winter day, while I stand on a bit of frozen earth in my backyard. I am a romantic and, like other romantics, I have trained myself to see beyond what my eyes tell me is there.

It is easy for me to go outside on a fine cold day like today and listen to the sound of honking geese as they fly overhead with me standing in the barren winter garden. The leaves of my emotions tremble at the sound and at the sight of these elegant birds. As they fade from sight, I hear in my head a whisper with a question, why do you garden? It is a question the unself-confident ask when the earth is hard, cold and unyielding. The question never occurred to me in over forty years of cultivating plants but suddenly I found it a mystery beyond poetry.

Such lonely thoughts can be dangerous in the emptiness of a winter garden, especially for someone who once thought of himself as tough-minded. There was exposed in the cold morning another, secret side to me, glimpsed rarely, those times when I went mushy at the sight of birds winging south for winter. My reaction to those moments was to purse my mouth and grit my teeth to prevent so much as a reflection of emotion from carousing across my face.

On this brittle cold afternoon, I feel on the verge of finding the answer to what turned me from being a muckraker into a muckworm. It was a notion flashed before me and I have always distrusted insight appearing as if it were a natural element. There it purred in the sun like a fat, happy cat: *gardening is a way to transcend everyday life.* It is a crazy thought, even for a guy who threw away his dog-eared catechism forty years ago when he broke ranks with the regiment.

To transcend life, garden. Could it be an idea stolen from Thoreau, the mystical naturalist of the New England woods?

Gardening transcends everyday life.

Was it an idea crossing the mind of old, grizzled Barbara Checco, the earthy-mouthed philosopher of the DeBiaggio clan? These were people with a peasant's straightforward gait. They went to the heart of the matter. It was Barbara Checco who told a friend's son who thought of his father as a god: "Don't think your father something supernatural, boy. He was the first Italian in Des Moines to have credit at all the whorehouses."

Everyday life can be transcended by gardening.

Now, here I was, a son of these people of the soil, in my backyard, tall and glorious, with my feet planted on hard Virginia clay, twitching with the idea that gardening is a means to transcend everyday life. Gardening may become a transcending experience but it does not transcend life. Gardening is as necessary as thinking and breathing because it is a reflection of life. Gardening teaches it is not necessary to transcend everyday life. Gardening exists to celebrate life every day.

*   *   *

SEPTEMBER 15, 1996

Dear Linda,

Cool weather has arrived. I was taking my daily three-mile walk about seven a.m. when a woman bundled in a cheap blue coat with a hood yelled at me from across Wilson Boulevard's four lanes. "Hey, mister, have you got any change," she hollered.

I crossed the street and opened my coin purse in her hands. She got everything, but it wasn't much, probably not enough for breakfast at the 7-Eleven outside of which she often sits in a sleeping bag. Many mornings I see men asleep on park benches with coats over them. One day there was a man curled up under a shrub beneath the window of an apartment.

These sights along my morning walk allow me to see how much things have changed in my hometown in the last fifty years. I remember a time before television when Mr. Rice next door chopped off a chicken's head and, from our window, I watched the dead bird jump involuntarily until it dropped and was picked and cleaned for Sunday afternoon dinner. It was a time when it was unusual for a family to have a car, and we massaged white margarine to make it yellow. An exciting Christmas in those days was receiving a set of wooden blocks your father made secretly in the shed out back. I thought there was plenty then, at least after World War II. We have so much more now, yet all of us don't seem to have enough.

Sometimes my life falls to the floor and I get down on my knees and grope for it in the dark.

*   *   *

Gardeners, like farmers, complain incessantly. Nothing appears to go right for them. If it's dry, they complain about drought. When it rains, they grouse about the loss of a crop to the flood. This trait is not uncommon outside the confederation of those who till the soil. Lawyers, doctors, presidents and laborers rant and shout over the inconsistencies of life, too. After a while, it can become an intolerable habit. I'm so contrary by nature and inclination I sometimes turn reality on its head capriciously. I've learned to make my bed but not to lie in it. To folks of this persuasion, life can seem harsh. They, as do I, rant a lot.

When ranting doesn't work, I find a good book and about thirty minutes, put on my spectacles and measure words carefully. A book I keep handy for such moments is *A Summer in the Garden,* an unregistered literary classic masquerading as garden writing. The wit, style and poetry of Charles Dudley Warner, the author, deserves some space in our modern psyches.

You can guess why I was drawn to it with writing like this: "The neighbors' small children are also out of place in your garden, in strawberry and currant time. I hope I appreciate the value of children. We should soon come to nothing without them. . . . But the problem is, what to do with them in a garden. For they are not good to eat, and there is a law against making away with them. The law is not very well enforced, it is true; for people do thin them out with constant dosing, paregoric, and soothing syrups, and scanty clothing. But I, for one, feel that it would not be right, aside from the law, to take the life, even of the smallest child, for the sake of a little fruit, more or less, in the garden. I may be wrong; but these are my sentiments and I am not ashamed of them. . . . My plan would be to put them into Sunday schools more thoroughly, and to give the Sunday schools an agricultural turn; teaching the children the sacredness of neighbors' vegetables. I think that our Sunday schools do not sufficiently impress upon children the danger, from snakes and otherwise, of going into the neighbors' gardens."

Warner was a man who found morals in the garden and related them with a wink: "You can tell when people are ripe by their willingness to let go. Richness and ripeness are not exactly the same. The rich are apt to hang to the stem with tenacity. I have nothing against the rich. If I were not virtuous, I should like to be rich. But we cannot have everything, as the man said when he was down with smallpox and cholera, and the yellow fever came into the neighborhood."

Like all gardeners Warner is philosophic about a common enemy: "By the time a man gets to be 80, he learns that he is compassed by limitations, and that there has been a natural boundary set to his individual powers. As he goes on in life, he begins to doubt his ability to destroy all evil and to reform all abuses, and to suspect that there will be much left to do after he has done. I stepped into my garden in the spring, not doubting that I should be easily master of the weeds. I have simply learned that an institution which is at least 6,000 years old, and I believe six millions, is not to be put down in one season."

When there are not weeds to be pulled there are nagging questions to answer: "I do not hold myself bound to answer the question, Does gardening pay? It is so difficult to define what is meant by paying. . . . As I look at it, you might as well ask, Does a sunset pay? I know that a sunset is commonly looked on as a cheap entertainment; but it is really one of the most expensive. It is true that we can all have front seats, and we do not exactly need to dress for it as we do for the opera; but the conditions under which it is to be enjoyed are rather dear. Among them I should name a good suit of clothes. . . . I should add also a good dinner, well cooked and digestible; and the cost of a fair education, extended, perhaps, through generations in which sensibility and love of beauty grew. What I mean is, that if a man is hungry and naked and half a savage, or with the love of beauty undeveloped in him, a sunset is thrown away on him: so that it appears that the conditions of the enjoyment of a sunset are as costly as anything in our civilization."

It must be quite clear by now that Charles Dudley Warner and I have so much in common that we might be family members; at the very least there are tribal similarities. We both celebrate life and gardening by ranting at inconveniences.

> I suppose I was not always what you call a Christian gentleman. My childhood filled me with dismay. I knew that Illinois was one of the richest and finest states in the Union; my father seldom said anything around the house, serving nearly twenty years in Sing-Sing for writing an out-spoken letter to a rear-Admiral. Mother had her points, never being able to get her weight up above sixty pounds. My brothers and sisters perished when someone carelessly left all the gas-jets open on the kitchen stove.
> —KENNETH PATCHEN, *Sleepers Awake*

SEPTEMBER 24, 1996

Dear Linda,

I am delighted you have the old ration book. Objects make for much stronger ties to the past and can serve to release powerful memories. My fondest relic is the ticket that brought my grandfather to America. It was found in my grandmother's safe deposit box after she died a few years ago. Although Grandpa always said the food on the ship was lousy, the menu on the back of the ticket doesn't sound bad. Like most food, and much of life, reality sometimes rests between expectations and execution.

On the surface, I am as calm as a cucumber and as sane as an apple. Inside, I'm the guy who gets anxious waiting for water from the faucet to turn hot. One spring, a bird changed my life a little.

In midspring that year, I found a little bundle of feathers in the driveway. It turned out to be soft and alive, a baby bird unable to fly, walk, or even sit up. It was helpless, hopeless and abandoned. It became my robin, if any wild creature can belong to anything or anybody.

There was an old nest in the bushes, vacated several years earlier by short-term tenants. I brought it around front and stuck it in the upper reaches of an upright yew next to the front steps. It was comical to see the baby robin hunkered down in the dried grass, twigs, string and plastic of the old nest.

Soon the responsibility of this find in the driveway descended upon me like a heavy weight. I wasn't a robin and I didn't have the slightest idea how to raise a baby bird. I searched for written advice in the library but there was no Dr. Spock for birds between hard covers.

Joyce saw my consternation, seized the moment, and in her direct way began telephoning naturalists, the zoo and animal welfare people. Finally, a voice on the phone offered hope. The voice suggested watered-down dog food as an appropriate meal for the robin.

I substituted chicken cat food, a supply of which was at hand, parceling it out with tweezers into the upturned beak of the robin. I tried to imitate the motion birds make in feeding their young. I held the tweezers high over the baby bird and made sharp little movements toward the baby's beak. I saw birds in National Geographic television specials do this. It worked and the little bird loved the cat food. But he was as messy as any child could be. I became worried about the need for toilet training.

After ten days of tweezers-feeding every daylight hour, the robin responded, putting on weight and color to his breast. He was active enough for a cat to notice. Into the greenhouse he went, safe, warm and with plenty of room to move about. A mascot for the greenhouse had arrived.

Once in the greenhouse, the robin did little flying. He hid under the benches and waited for me to come out the kitchen door and dash for the greenhouse, chicken cat food can in one hand, tweezers in the other.

"Robbie, Robbie," I called to the bird.

The little robin half flew, half danced across the dirt to me. He stood at my feet and flapped his wings madly, anticipating a good meal. The diet also became more varied; I began to dig an occasional worm, and cherries were ripe on the tree in the backyard. The robin grew with amazing speed; his orange breast developed spots, the sign of an immature bird, and he was almost full size.

Robbie became more than a bird in a greenhouse. He was a charming mascot and friend who listened intently. When it came time to water plants, he followed me up and down the rows between the benches, coming dangerously close to my feet. He danced in the water draining through the pots. What a joy he became.

One morning I decided it was time to release the bird. Robbie had become too dependent on the man who couldn't care for him forever. It was a sad morning. I choked with emotion, and tears puffed my eyes. I was emotionally attached to a bird.

In the vast scheme of things, releasing a captive robin is a small event. In my small world it was momentous. I held the robin on my trembling index finger as I had so many times, but we were outside this time. The robin clung to my finger for dear life. He wasn't about to fly away willingly. A catbird perched on the telephone wires overhead screamed at the man with the bird balancing on his forefinger. Finally, I touched the bird softly, caressing it in both hands and gently tossed him toward the sky. He soared for a moment and was over the high wooden fence on which the rosebush climbs. Robbie was gone, released after a meal of chicken cat food, into a world full of hazards. I was alone and almost beside myself with depression. My wild friend was gone.

Would Robbie learn the necessary safety techniques fast enough to survive? Could a bird brought up to meow survive in an urban jungle of marauding cats, bicyclists, automobiles, airplanes and pollution? I remembered reading that 80 percent of all baby robins die before reaching maturity. Do mothers all feel the way I did as their offspring march off to fulfill themselves in the world?

For hours, I was mush and my eyes misty. I couldn't take a deep breath without the air trembling in my throat and my eyes filling with tears. Would I ever see my feathered friend again? Would I ever witness the feeding ritual in which the robin flapped his wings and stretched his neck up with mouth wide open and made little giggling sounds as the tweezers holding the cat food approached?

When we lose something special like this, we gain in humanity and the world changes just a little for us and for those we meet. It makes us richer than we can possibly be any other way. It helps sweeten our sourness.

Around lunchtime, I was crossing the patio when I looked up into the cherry tree. There, dancing through the limbs, was Robbie.

"Robbie, Robbie," I called to him.

The bird swooped down to my shoulder. It was feeding time and Robbie was anxious about his next meal. I moved the robin to another greenhouse in which the bird could get in and out by himself through roof vents. Robbie hid under the benches and pecked at the soft dirt. He still followed me as I watered the plants, enjoying water dripped through the pots.

The bird, in the manner of robins everywhere, liked to walk around outside the protective greenhouse. One morning as I watered in the greenhouse, Robbie took a walk on the gravel path opposite me. The bird sauntered down the path toward the old Spanish sundial, when out of the corner of my eye I saw a cat lying in wait. The cat pounced, a streak of gray shooting out of green boxwood leaves. Feathers flew everywhere. Robbie soared into the air and perched on the ridge of the greenhouse out of harm's way, no worse for the experience. It was a close call; too close, I thought. The nursery was no place for a too-tame robin.

I found the old bamboo birdcage in the attic, put the robin in it, and headed for Potomac Overlook Regional Park. The park has acres of undisturbed woods and hugs the Potomac River just down from Great Falls where the fresh water froths over rocks in its slow, determined course to the salty Atlantic Ocean. There are hundreds of robins in this park and I took Robbie to a little grassy place where I saw robins pull fat, red worms out of the ground. I reached into the cage and took the bird out carefully and placed him on the grass. I stood up and watched the bird hop around on the soft, green grass for a moment. I backed away with the birdcage in my hand. The air caught in my throat and the tears sprinted down my cheeks.

Suddenly, the bird soared into the air and flew into the trees. It was the last time I saw him.

I returned to search through the woods for a speckle-breasted young robin who would answer to the name Robbie. I felt foolish calling his name. Wild things do not have names and the bird was wild now as surely as the wind is wild and untamed. The wild should remain ungoverned and unkept, but I will always cherish those few late spring weeks when Robbie and I were together like brothers, when we had so much to learn about each other and about ourselves in the world.

Cats with their soft, colorful fur are silent menders of time and memory.

*   *   *

The gypsy knew ahead of time
Our secret night-imprisoned lives
We said good-bye to her and hope
sprang without reason from that well.
Love like a ponderous trained bear
Danced upright in our slightest will
The blue-bird lost his lovely plumes
And all the mendicants their beads.
We knew that we had damned ourselves
But hope which beckoned there
Made us think hand in hand of what
The gypsy had foretold for us.

— NEW DIRECTIONS,
The Selected Writings of Apollinaire

As WINTER WANES and weather warms, the fish become alive as they float to the top of the water and dive into dark places. The koi leap over each other hungrily to reach the rough, brown pellets I throw into the cold March water. It is a marker of the warm times ahead.

Hide me. Hold me. Never let me go.

March is a month of great promise, but it is still too cold to offer much return from the garden. Spring can be felt in the sun's warmth when days are noticeably longer. The high school students who start their days early, along with me, no longer have to walk in the dark to school. At this latitude, March is the most important month for the rest of the season in the herb garden. On the deeds done now rest future growth and harvest.

March is also a month in which to make inquiries of the garden and its inhabitants. What has made it through the winter?

It is a constant question asked of plants not yet outfitted for spring. Is it dead? That's the question when staring at the ground covered with the brown, dry straw that were last year's herbs. Did that plant make it through the winter? How much of it survived? Bare, woody branches, dried leaves rattling in the wind, vacant ground where once the garden flourished. Spring on the verge is an anxious time.

March also brings more to do than worry about what's alive and what's dead. Clearing the debris and pulling the ever-present winter crop of chickweed is a continual task. Other cleanup chores also await: cutting back last year's now-dead stalks of tarragon and oregano, removing dead wood from the thyme and sage and then pruning it back low to the ground so it doesn't get woody and keeps its hungry vigor. In youth, as in spring, it is well to assess the present and look to the future. The discipline of regular chores, performed with attention and care, helps to calm early anxieties and convince the mind all is well and life is secure.

A shadow as thin as a slice of tomorrow follows me around. It is the memory of yesterday.

AFTER ROBBIE DISAPPEARED on his soft, young feathers into the deep, shaded woods of Algonquin Park high above the Potomac, I continued to return to the place, foolish enough to think he might recognize me. Of course I was just another trespasser to a bird, and to my consternation I was an interloper and not a friend.

The trees were high and dense and even during the day, at ground level, it was always near dark in the leafy bower. I took these walks through the woods on Sunday mornings when the earth was still and I could listen to myself without distraction. It was here I began jotting down thoughts that bubbled to my brain as I walked over rough, sloping terrain.

There were always leaves littering the path and in the fall they were crisp and it was hard to be silent. Here I could hear nature breathe softly and inhale the rich scents coming from surprising places along the well-worn clay path. There were other things new to me and their names are secret to this day. I took photos of some of these hidden wonders. One was a picture of moss in bloom. The photo is taken at ground level and above the mound of green moss it appears the sky is on fire.

A second photo shows the morning haze as the sun bursts through, showing the dark shapes of bare tree trunks as the fallen leaves scurry toward the light.

In another, a parade of white umbrella mushrooms staggers along against a dark almost purple background of decaying leaves. Just below it, already in action, is a young deer, leaving no shape, only its movement as it runs away.

Another photo shows a deer who has turned and begins to run. From the rear she appears to be wearing a white boa.

My favorite is a photo in a dense part of the little forest on a frosty morning with scant visibility. A blue shroud hangs against a background of stately trees while a busy wind lifts the dying leaves from their attachment to a thick grove of trees.

During one visit, I was able to photograph a lovely young deer standing in a mist of falling leaves.

My walk through the woods usually took about forty minutes on Sundays. Those walks were the closest I have been to church since I was sixteen.

The air was blank as it swirled into a killer breeze, whipped by a shower of small snow balls. A strange day for late March.

*   *   *

One calm evening as I made dinner, there were three powerful explosions, sending me into darkness. I saw fire leap from the power line across 10th Street next to the used car lot. The explosions left me breathless, as if my chest had been hit by a projectile. Electricity flicked off and on for a few moments before it went into darkness. The fire engines were on their way from the station house two blocks away. Rush-hour traffic was backed up as the fire crews blocked the street and waited for the power company crews to arrive.

WHEN I WAS YOUNG, I wore a rug of whiskers on my face and was cynical and inscrutable. Now, with age and the desire to shave every morning, I have become transparent, the original Cockeyed Optimist. Yet, I am still twisted by moods. As I sat on my haunches in the garden the other day diddling a little thyme plant, I felt a cloud pass over my face. Inscrutability returned with another spring.

I thought Robbie might have returned by now. My eyes were watery from the memories of the time I spent raising the robin.

I don't know why I thought Robbie might return, but humans need such events (they're often termed miracles by the religious). The whole idea of a robin swooping down on my shoulder to rekindle old times was foolish, but I needed a sign like the bird's return to acknowledge I played a useful and important part in Nature. Who would have thought soft feathers could turn my head and my heart so irrationally?

At six-thirty A.M. I came through the door carrying the newspaper. It was a bright June morning and I was smiling, but tears dripped down my cheeks.

"Robbie's back," I said softly to myself, struggling to make words fit through a constricted windpipe. There was no one else to hear the words. There are many things in life to make an otherwise sane man crazy. Not since St. Francis has a bird been known to be one of them.

The bird flew into an early-morning maple tree next door as I walked down the front stone steps. I watched intently and saw the robin hop up to the wiry curb of a nest and place a worm in an upturned beak.

I surprised myself. Instead of feeling foolish talking to a bird, I felt like a St. Francis. It was then I realized what the story of St. Francis is really about. It is a fanciful way to acknowledge our kinship with the wild. Did it matter whether this robin was last spring's memory of Robbie? I had to see Robbie again to make the folktale come true. The robin I raised the year before returned to show me that Nature was benevolent and needed me.

I sat down in front of the kitchen counter, leaving the paper in its blue plastic wrapper. I peeled an apple and ate it carefully. I thought about a bird talking to a man. It was then I decided not to mention it to anyone else. It was like keeping a mistress, a secret hidden from the world, a joy to be shared by two people.

The next morning I stole out the front door as the weak morning light peeked through leafy maple trees. I looked down the street, holding my breath, looking for the same experience of the previous morning. The robin was there again. Breathlessly, I approached the bird. The robin danced along the grass for a moment and then soared up to the cable television wire. He perched there and looked down at me as he had before.

"Robbie, Robbie," I called in a whisper. I called again louder. The robin cocked his head as if listening carefully, sorting out sounds. Then it flew away without a peep.

I was heartsore. I tried again the next morning, but I couldn't find the bird, it vanished like an apparition. Where once there was happiness and hope, there was now a hole reeking of remembered sadness. The seasons repeat but they are never the same.

*   *   *

Many of my plants look dead this spring, something I didn't expect from this winter. As the days warm and awaken what is left on the bushes and trees, I see the possibility of turning death into an act of life. It is a strange notion for even an old poet struggling with his mortality and the cloak of darkness.

Old men reach for another beer as winter sun warms their backs. Down the street dust rises above a falling office building. All around me devastation walks the streets, bumper to bumper in impatient cars.

❧

THERE WAS PLEASURE from bay trees (*Laurus nobilis*) for many years, but the fun did not become intense until my five 10-foot-high twelve-year-olds were threatened with extinction.

I dismantled the greenhouse in which the bays resided and faced a choice to chop them into sweet kindling or find a way to save them in an inhospitable climate without a greenhouse.

I was attached emotionally to these plants, a hopeless situation for a gardener. Emotion often makes humans silly, violent or confused. The thought of losing my bays did all three to me, but more than emotion was at stake. My laurels were money in the bank for me because I used them to produce rooted cuttings to grow into plants I sold.

Bay trees are easily grown from seed, I was assured by Otto Richter, the late prince of Canadian herb growers. So I did as he suggested and ordered a kilo of seeds. The seeds are a little larger than a green pea with a hard shell. They have a deserved reputation for being hard to germinate.

Before long there were 800 little bays with skinny, dark mahogany stems and green leaves. It was then I began to have the most fun. Not all seedlings looked alike. There were differences in leaf size and shape. Some without green leaves sported variegated leaves splashed with gold. Others looked like albinos with creamy leaves with red veins.

The bewildering array of bay variations amongst my seedlings was not unusual, I discovered later. An elderly gardener, a *paesano* from Pennsylvania who obtained bay seeds on a trip home to Italy, recounted a story similar to mine. Eli Putievsky, an Israeli herb researcher, surveyed the wild population of bays in a native habitat in the northern mountains of his country and discovered twenty-one distinct varieties. The Israeli bays had heavy concentrations of large, dark green leaves along the stems while others were sparsely filled; some trees were tall and others were short. The plant's essential oil also varied. One of Putievsky's finds had a "good lemony" aroma; another, a medium-sized tree with very large leaves, was almost without aroma.

I moved the large bays into tubs eighteen inches high and twenty-four inches in diameter. They weighed 150 pounds each. I didn't have the heart to throw them away. The sensible thing to do was to hold them until I could plant them and let nature take care of them. Winter temperatures here in Virginia often tumble below zero, killer territory for bay.

By October, the hot days disappeared and temperatures moderated enough to move the bays from tubs into deep holes sheltered by the south side of the house. Winter hit before I could spray them with a protectant to prevent winter dehydration. As the icy winds howled in December, I wrapped them in cones of Microfoam, a closed-cell poly product used to overwinter nursery stock. The lush green bay trees vanished into huge white stalagmites thrusting toward the winter sky.

When spring arrived, I unwrapped the bays. I was almost in tears when I saw the damage winter left: split bark and dry, brown leaves. The experiment appeared to have failed, but I couldn't bear to remove them. I left them to mock me.

As I raked the debris created by the bays' dead leaves several months later, I saw red shoots sprouting from the bay roots. The roots in the sun-warmed earth survived. By summer's end, my bays were just over four feet, half their original height.

Bay laurels may have a fickle heart, but they gave me a new understanding of nature and myself. Just when I thought I understood a lot, the garden wiggled my confidence and opened my eyes to the pleasures of taking chances.

Scattered words, lost in a low land, wander through brocaded memories. A world once known hides behind a gauze of bewilderment. Sparkling eyes dim.

EUROPEANS HAVE A demonstrated knack for commercializing wild plant populations. The French lavender industry began by gathering and drying wild lavender and steaming the essential oils from the freshly cut wild flowers.

The Portuguese permit jays to scatter oak acorns across the landscape and then strip the bark from the adult trees every nine years to produce cork. The process is somewhat inefficient by industrial standards but it beats even no-till agriculture.

At night I hear the darkness in my ears as I try to sleep. During the day the cars swish along the busy streets. I saw something of air and silence this afternoon under the bright sun. It was time for hurry in clusters as the cars headed for home and away from offices.

An acquaintance dedicated to thyme told me once he feared his neighbors were wondering about his sanity.

Every spring, he said, he took wheelbarrows of gravel up the hill to the thyme bed and worked it into the soil to improve the drainage for his collection. These small stones were also useful to mulch plants, although it turned out mulch failed to tame the summer explosion of weeds.

His care seemed quite logical to me. I read research reporting that an inch or two of sand spread as a mulch on the soil beneath lavender plants lessened disease, prevented winter loss and provided plants with greater harvests. There was also some research suggesting wood chips used as a mulch around basil plants lessened the debilitating effects of *erwinia,* a disease causing stem discoloration, leaf wilt and eventually death.

My friends' fixation with gravel was matched by my own quirky passion, altering my hard, unyielding clay soil with what surely must now be tons of humus, mostly in the form of peat moss. I realized that both of us, in our dedication to improving the life of our plants, may have slipped off the level plane other mortals maintained.

He who says herbs are carefree plants of easy cultivation has spent more time in the library than in the garden. One year I toured herb gardens connected with some of the cultural shrines of California. I saw dryness in the south, a perfect climate for herbs. I looked carefully and saw many of the same problems I have in my East Coast backyard. I came away with the realization that the same problems inhabited the West Coast as the humid East Coast.

Herbs can sometimes be extraordinarily easy, especially when they self-sow in the garden. When I first grew dill and chamomile, the plants threw seeds all over and every year dill and chamomile weeds germinate regularly. Parsley and coriander often do the same in the garden.

Some gardeners actually buy purslane seed and grow it in their gardens. Purslane is a delightful salad green used by people with more refined tastes than mine, but the plant has grown on my small part of the earth for more than twenty years despite my vigorous weeding and shows no signs of going away.

I remember a glorious stand of borage one year from seeds someone gave me after a lecture. They were a rare, white-flowered variety gathered in France. The flowers *were* white but they were very late and minuscule, and hardly noticeable among the fat leaves. I forgot to gather the seed and trusted it would self-sow, but no white-flowered borage came up the next year.

Usually, self-sown seed comes up around where the parent was. This is quite understandable, but why is a blue-flowered borage sprouting in the gravel seventy-five feet from where its parent was last year? Self-sown plants make sowing seeds look easy. It makes you wonder why there are so many books on the subject and so many complaints by gardeners that they "have no luck with seeds."

A gauze of perdition hangs from what was once a fine cherry tree. Now a scruffy obelisk is tattered and lifeless, waiting for a stiff wind to blow it away.

When I set out for a trip to the store, I have something in mind to buy. When I reach my destination, there is a blank spot where there was a message. I don't know why I am there and I get in the car empty-handed and head home. One day I will lose my way home and stop driving forever.

I am a slow learner. It's taken me nearly half a century to comprehend that there is more to medicine than sticking a thermometer under your tongue when you feel bad. I have John Victor to thank for a splint on my fractured medical education.

Victor, a former neighbor, is an enthusiastic jumble of a man with a passion for herbs and books. He showed up one warm, spring day with a dog-eared antique, a thin, now unbound book by Benjamin Shultz.

In 1795, Shultz published this little treatise and called it *On the Phytolacca decandra of Linnaeus*. It was subtitled *Botanical-*

Medical Dissertation. The book's publication was, according to Victor, the final step for Shultz to become a medical practitioner.

The *Phytolacca decandra* of the book's title, as I discovered with a little botanical research, is now called *Phytolacca americana,* a plant known commonly as poke. *Hortus,* often considered to be the bible of horticultural botany, says it is an herb growing to twelve feet "with an unpleasant odor and large poisonous root." Unknown to anonymous *Hortus* authors is this vigorous weed's penchant for growing next to the beautiful Golden Showers rose in my garden. Poke has a taproot nearly impossible to eradicate in such a position.

So, here was Dr. Shultz, a member of the Philadelphia Medical Society, singing the therapeutic praises of pokeweed. I dove into the book with an abandon usually reserved for sexy potboilers.

The dissertation began with an idea frequently expressed today. "With what enthusiasm," wrote Shultz, "and at how much expense, do we send many thousand miles for exotic plants, whose virtues may, perhaps, be far inferior to many of our own, which, by a little industry, might be brought to a state of culture and perfection, of which other countries cannot boast, and of which preceding botanists have had but faint idea!"

Poke, for Dr. Shultz, was just such a plant, an abundant, native weed he thought might cure cancer, rheumatism, gout, dysentery and syphilis. This miracle remedy was easy to rationalize. Dr. Shultz believed that "all the variety of universal diseases which we meet with at different times, are originally but one and the same disease, viz. a fever."

I thumbed the yellowing pages with mounting wonder. Spread before me was a record by an enthusiastic young doctor of a series of experiments on himself and his little dog using different parts of the plant. The ingestion of tinctures of leaf and root, or of dark purple berry juice, always appeared to have the same effect: prolonged vomiting.

"I believe the *Phytolacca* will never prove fatal as a narcotic," Shultz wrote in a footnote, "because when given in large doses, it will always procure its own rejection by its emetic power."

I had to put the book aside for a moment to calm my stomach. These eighteenth-century folk seem to have spent a great deal of time puking to get well. They raised it to one of their medical arts, along with bloodletting.

The Good Doctor Shultz was more than two centuries before his time in at least one way. He anticipated complaints by activists about medical experiments on animals. The mongrel who retched so much for him after swallowing his pokeweed concoctions benefitted from the experiments, according to Shultz. When he "procured" the animal, the dog "was very scabby," he wrote in a footnote, "but after the experiments were concluded, he was perfectly cured."

Shultz noted a bit of history in passing, a salient comment on his times. Portuguese and French wine makers used the dark purple juice squeezed from poke berries (the plant is also indigenous to Europe) in red wine as an adulterant to darken the grape juice. Of course, the adulterated wine made people sick. Louis XVI banned the practice and instituted the death penalty for any wine maker caught poking wine. Making people sick from poke juice became the sole province of doctors.

I have tried to uphold the old European garden traditions of my great-grandfather, Domenico DeBiaggio, and his brother, Francesco, and let no grass grow on my 5,000-square-foot lot. I have also tried to follow the catechism set down by those two grand old gardeners and make every inch of my garden productive.

Horticultural productivity does not come easily when faced with sticky, orange Virginia clay whose most common use is brick making, not agriculture. To change the soil's productivity, I learned early to alter its complexion, and I added copious amounts of humus to create dark, fertile mounds. Despite my eagerness to kill grass to create fertile soils, I continue to be nagged by the feeling to do better, get a little more out of the dirt, use the space more profitably.

You can understand my surprise and relief when I discovered two Italian parsley plants growing from the cracks in the mortar of the brick steps descending from my house into the backyard. I was surprised these plants found a site on their own and made use of a bit of space I overlooked. The spirits of Meni and Checco hovering over my garden saw to what lengths I followed their peasant dictates to use all available space for food.

It amused me to watch these parsley plants struggle to grow without my help in this hard, barren brick garden. In a fit of inexplicable distemper, brought about by my proclivity to get everything neat and tidy for winter, I yanked the parsley plants, threw them out, and put an end to their struggle and, I thought, to all green things sprouting from cracks in mortar and bricks.

My amusement with the parsley turned into a newfound humility the next spring. A small alpine strawberry plant sprouted where the parsley plants were once. It grew almost unnoticed until it flowered and produced a small crop of red berries. It was then I inspected the strawberry carefully and found an oregano seedling growing underneath it. The oregano was a small, hard specimen difficult to identify, but close to *Origanum majoricum,* a hybrid unlikely to have viable seed. My wonder at this botanical marvel before me deflected my thoughts momentarily from the strawberry, but the ripening berries reminded me of future pleasures.

This unexpected garden growing from brick steps was the perfect place to confuse birds who ate these tiny strawberries just before full ripening. It was easy to confuse the birds, which were more interested in the ripening cherries on a nearby tree. Slugs are lazy and opportunistic and they stayed interested in a pot of zinnias at the foot of the steps. I had the pleasure one cool June morning to eat a succulent, perfume-sweet strawberry from the plant growing out of the brick steps. It was a strawberry whose taste was as perfect as one carefully cultivated.

Simple things count: a cat playing with a shadow cast by an open window, a piece of wild twine blowing on the windowsill.

WHEN I WAS a wee lad, I had a small, black cocker pup named Inky. As the owner of Man's Best Friend, I looked upon cats and their benefactors with disdain. It was an attitude rather than a belief, as are so many things in life. Even at so young an age, you could see the man forming in the child.

There was only one dog in my life and every minute of Inky was beautiful, especially the energetic pup racing after me and grabbing my pants' cuff. Such affection could not last.

As I developed an inner anger at the world, and the little black dog fattened with age, we grew apart. When I left home, the dog stayed behind and, I am ashamed to say, I felt not a twinge of emotion. I steeled myself with a scowl and a frown, and pretended to feel only biological urges.

With some maturity, I discovered cats were furry, bright predators with a cantankerous side. They were individualistic to a fault. I thought I saw a wink of myself in cats' behavior toward the world.

As I grew older, I fell in love with a cat fancier smitten with the idea of a cat sitting on her lap and purring. Eventually a son was born and a cat was added along with a baby stroller. Unfortunately, the little cat died before it was a year old. I didn't have much reaction to the kitten's death. I was still a long way from the time when the earth's sharp edges became dull and I permitted myself a twinge of emotion from time to time.

Much later I fell madly in love with a slightly used pair of part Himalayan cats, fuzzy, beautiful and with smoky dark markings around the face. They were already over a year old and set in their ways when the advertisement offering them to a good home was answered. Joyce and I picked them up one afternoon from their former keeper and dropped them off at our house on our way to some special event.

When we returned, our new cats were nowhere to be seen and remained so for several days. Frightened into silence and scared of the new surroundings, the two cats hid in places inaccessible to humans until they were discovered. It was an inauspicious beginning to a love affair lasting over fifteen joyful years.

These were not lap cats, if there are such things except in dreams, and they acted out their new names, Prince and Princess. They were like all cats in my life—they received everything they desired. It never appeared they were demanding anything. When these cats got their way and purred, it was as if they were saying, "I will love you forever."

When anybody has been around cats for a short while, they think they know them. I knew nothing. Prince and Princess demanded a certain brand of canned cat food and of that brand a special meal: chicken, always the same chicken. If I wanted to vary the menu, the cats rebelled and walked away with what the French might call *hauteur*. There was no way to nudge these unadventurous felines toward an appreciation of the tasty variety of life.

Other cats showed varying degrees of this single-mindedness about food. Nifty, my son's cat, was the most easily pleased, when he ate at all. Sam, a neighborhood stray with a sweet temper and a loud purr-box, seemed fixated on squirrel; he ate everything but tail and claws.

My latest feline guests are the most peculiar of any I have ever known. We call them Una and Sabina. Una is an inquisitive, All-American, striped cat with subtle shades of gray and brown. Sabina has a smoke body with a dark mask and the volubility and tone of a Siamese. They are both girls, unrelated, and both with checkered pedigrees. Did you know a cat can give birth to a single litter of kittens that have different fathers? Sabina and the vet taught me that. Life remains interesting even when the soaps aren't flickering across the television screen.

These two cats are sweet and playful. These are inside cats, knowing nothing of the outside world beyond what they see through the windows at which they perch expectantly at sunrise and sunset. This way of feline life may seem cruel to some cat lovers, but it is better than scraping road-kill cats off the street.

One morning I looked up from the breakfast newspaper and found Una in the kitchen sink eating the pulp and seeds left from a cantaloupe. From then on, both cats insisted each morning on cantaloupe. I obliged them with paper-thin fillets of the fruit chopped ever so small on separate plates. One morning the cantaloupe was a shade unripe; both cats refused the fillets and left the kitchen in a huff.

The taste for cantaloupe was only the beginning of the cats' romp through the gourmet's life. Somehow or other Una convinced me she needed some grass to munch. How she realized it was missing from her diet is only one part of the mystery. Now I go to the garden every summer morning to pick from an assortment of green weeds flourishing there.

Una waits by the door expectantly when I return and as soon as she sees the green bouquet, she rises on her hind legs and extends her front paws to accept the gift. The bouquet goes into a glass of water and Una begins munching on the green stuff. Soon Sabina gets wind of the booty and joins in with less gusto, as is her hesitant style.

After the two kittens have gorged themselves, they lie satiated on the living room rug in the sunshine. I inspect the bouquet. Both cats have selectively passed up the Bermuda grass and the real grass. Una and Sabina have a taste for crabgrass, especially the young weed not yet in seed.

So, now each morning when I come in the house after my before-breakfast inspection of the greenhouse, Una waits for the green bouquet of fresh crabgrass which she shares with Sabina while they await the cantaloupe fillets.

The romance and mystery of history did not clothe my weeds when I first saw them begin to sprout in the freshly turned soil. I perceived them as nuisances then, and not as living artifacts. In those long-ago days, I became churlish easily and weeds were to blame.

Several decades ago, in a little hospital in Hardin County, Iowa, I watched my mother die slowly of cancer. Her once luminous skin gradually turned green from the disease as she wasted away weak and alone.

The hospital room was big and contained two beds and a large window through which light poured early in the morning. A nurse asked me if I wanted to sleep the night there in the spare bed, as my sister had earlier, but I was so uncomfortable in the presence of death I could not.

My mother lay on her side most of the time. She was quiet and the only sound between us often was her quiet breathing. Occasionally, she looked over at me sitting in a chair and struggled to smile. She could no longer eat but occasionally her arm ventured slowly from the sheet covering her and her hand plucked a chip of ice from a bowl beside her. She sucked the ice carefully, with great concentration. There was not much left for either of us to say and, yet, too much needed saying. Being quiet together sufficed.

Her death came before it was time, as had my father's four years earlier. It came too early for her and for me. A young man's experience cannot prepare him for such events and simple words lay silent in my mouth.

The scars borne by the survivors of those who die young are invisible but they are rough and deep, and just when you think they have healed, the tears come in a flood.

These memories and events encircled me many years later as I struggled to bring silent seeds to life in a late winter, dark with overcast skies. Many times have I made metaphor, comparing the seasons of the garden with life and death. On days when I touch soft earth and hard seed, I often remember the slow agony of a woman dying in a little hospital in Hardin County, Iowa. It was then I first questioned the ability of words to quiet the raw emotions engendered by death.

We can understand life through the metaphor of gardens. During winter the ground is muddy, frozen and barren; for all the world it appears dead and useless. When the warmth and long days of summer arrive, the garden, planted with fresh plump vegetables, graceful flowers and scented herbs, is vibrantly full of life.

In life, as in the garden, the dark secret of unpredictable death puzzles and bewilders, intrigues and frightens. Everyone reaches to touch the newborn child and hold its promise of young, long life, but at the same time, we wish the elderly out of sight; their wrinkles and infirmities remind us of what awaits for them and for us.

In life there are sweet and glorious revelations every day, but the deep secrets hidden by death, especially that of a relative or dear friend, remain unknown and as mysterious as the fog.

When I dug my first garden, I found a backyard full of artifacts as solid as concrete and as fragile as glass bottles. I also unearthed objects too small to see, but they soon made themselves noticed. These tiny objects were seeds, and some of them may have been snuggled underground for fifty years or more, waiting for me to come along and treat them to a bit of wake-up sunshine.

As magnificent as was this miracle of long-delayed germination, I summed up the little plants the seeds made in one bitter
word: weeds. I have pulled these weeds, and their offspring, for
nearly thirty years and I am sure others before me did the same
in fruitless, but divine labor.

Only recently has it occurred to me that many of my
actions have become ritualized. Along with this I see
many of my thoughts have a finality to them. The room I
live in is shrinking as I float along toward death. Dreams
are disappearing. The doors are closing. The days are not
long enough.

❋

THE GREENHOUSE, not empty but deserted during the day, has
no place of its own in the backyard. I abandoned it sometime
ago in a flood of tears and fear. For many years, this place was a
happy, throbbing zone of happy faces. The work was hard but
rewarding. The large structure remains to ignite memories
from me and others. Birds fly between steel beams crisscrossing
the upper reaches of the open roof.

This big, brooding structure is in the way, but I still want it
where it is. Despite its size and decrepit appearance, it remains
because Alzheimer's is destroying my brain, losing all that matters in my world. I want things like the greenhouse to remind
me of who I am and where I have been, a touchstone of a fast-
fading past.

I want to touch the greenhouse with my eyes and stroke it
like one of my cats. I want to watch how quickly the tactile
touch runs to memory and retrieves a scene glazed in time, a
picture from an old photo in my Grandma Davis's stereopticon.

I stand in my little workroom, papers littering the desk
behind me, waiting for the moment of enlightenment on a

sunny day in February. I look down on the greenhouse covering most of the backyard. The roof is full of sun this bright February day. To the left, over the fence, two men wash cars, part of a rental operation. Inside the greenhouse, a jumble of plants have lingered too long, waiting for the compost pile.

As I look down on this piece of my history, I cannot bring a tear to my eyes. The greenhouse is an image of me, now distressed, lingering, with a stack of pills in the kitchen cabinet. We are both on our last days, but still useful.

Inside the greenhouse there is chaos. The steel bench tops are filled with dead plants caught in a sudden cold spell. The greenhouse was not enough to protect its subjects without heat and I forgot to turn it on. There is a scent of death here, even as sunlight pours through the open roof vents. I look over the large outside room and see myself with disheveled mind to match the carelessness of this place that has meant so much to me over so many years. Neither I nor the greenhouse has much to hide. Both of us have slippery memories to explore.

You are familiar but I don't remember your name.

❦

I MADE TWO trips to Iowa as summer sputtered into fall; one to say goodbye to the enduring matriarch of the DeBaggio family, my 104-year-old grandmother, Lottie; and a second trip six weeks later to bury her.

The four grandchildren who survive her are completely on their own, having lost their parents decades ago, their grandfather, and now this wise, reassuring woman whose life spanned the turbulence and promise of two centuries. Times like these test what is best in us, and true, and we see ourselves in the context of our remembered past and imagined future.

Word of my grandmother's death came in darkness with the

bleep of the phone. It was five A.M. and a woman filled with kindness and bewildered by details told me Grandma DeBaggio stopped breathing in her sleep during the night at the nursing home in Eldora, Iowa, where she lived her last years.

Within hours Joyce began to rummage through boxes of photographs and letters to seek clues to our life and Grandma's. We quickly sought to recapture a past now slipped from memory. We found little in the old boxes, but as we pried further, the past began to take shape differently than I remembered it.

Kind, wonderful Joyce handed me photographs and letters from a time my memory told me was a blistering emotional moment of moral torment, but the memories in these old boxes were not the chronicle of alienation I thought were there. The only remnants of the past to be felt and touched showed a non-violent struggle in our family to see each other as human beings. This was in the most difficult times of our lives, the sixties and seventies, when America swirled in moral chaos.

These were times ripping at our lives. These were times eating at our inner selves. These were times of division, alienation, war and deceit, leaving our emotions in shreds. Only the earth and time have the power to restore stillness. This was a time before the earth reached up to me through my garden and said, yes, it is all right to cry.

The present appears full of portents and small epiphanies when someone of your flesh and blood dies. As I prepared to leave for the funeral, I opened my *New York Times* to a review by Vincent Canby of a festival of films by Federico Fellini, the Italian movie maker whose images molded my late adolescent and early adult imagination. The review contained the first news this movie magician was near death.

"Toward the end of 'Voices of the Moon' (1990), Federico Fellini's latest film," Canby wrote, "there's a scene of incredible beauty and sadness. An angry old man named Gonnella, played by an actor who has something of the look and shape of a caricature of Fellini, enters a noisy disco and starts cursing the hedonistic dancers from a platform high above.

"He shouts into the din: 'Barbarians! Have you never heard the sound of a violin?' The people below stop and stare up at Gonnella. 'Dancing,' he says, 'should be like lace.' With that, he makes his way down to the dance floor. Taking the hand of his ancient mistress, he begins an elegant waltz. As he and the woman move gracefully around the floor, seeming to float on air, the old man hangs onto a life in which music, dance, and all the other arts still count for something.

"What the disco audience suspects, but Gonnella doesn't, is that he is quite dead. It's just that he refuses to lie down."

I left for Iowa with Canby's image from the Fellini film in mind. Is it possible to live so long the present is no longer understandable? My grandmother had an extraordinary memory and she recited poems from her school days, but she did not live in the past; the present animated her. She told me she lived too long, outlived too many generations of friends. Until she lost her hearing, and her eyesight dimmed, she kept up with the excitement of politics, science and books with remarkable savvy.

I am now at an age at which I can appreciate my grandmother's delight and wonder at the present, but I can also sympathize with Gonnella, for whom time passed so rapidly it became difficult to recognize the present as the child of the past. My grandmother never lost sight of the connection between past and present.

In early November, on my last visit to Eldora, I walked every morning through darkness to the bluff on the edge of town. It looks down on the Iowa River and holds in the rich darkness of its black earth the bodies of my family. I strolled through this silent community of marble and granite each morning as dawn approached. I stared down on the headstones of my father and mother and saw rosy, polished granite as the first light broke the darkness. I said nothing as I looked down on the stones carefully carved with their names, but the sight of these immobile granite markers in the brisk, cold dawn never failed to bring tears to my eyes, tears that did not come in an earlier time.

Those who have shed such tears know these are not tears of sadness, but tears of renewal, and when dampness on cheeks dries there is a wonderful clean feeling of joy in the body. I told no one of this experience, especially the kind strangers, Dorothy and Bill Bruner, who took me in, gave me their bed to sleep in, fed me, and made me feel as if I had known them a lifetime.

On a September morning in Eldora before I returned home, the last day I saw my grandmother alive, I decided to take a dawn tour of all the places she lived. As I walked in the darkness down strange streets, dogs barked and I wondered what it was I thought I could find of myself here in the place where I was born, or of her, other than the shriveled body lying in the nursing home bed breathing hard and anxiously. I walked past Happy Joe's where my cousin, Suzanna, and I took Grandma in a wheelchair for pizza the day before, and I realized I sought revelation in the old facades of Eldora.

As the golden light of dawn crept over the town, I knew by living long and doing much in her quiet way, my grandmother left an imprint on the town, and on the world, and on her grandchildren. What I saw in those old doorways to the past, and in those floating memories, was a legacy of hard work, generosity, and forgiveness that might warm us in our lives and in the lives that follow ours.

Funerals are full of sadness and tears, but they also have their share of hope and surprises. They remind us a rivulet of sorrow trickles through our lives to nourish the joys and triumphs.

I shut my eyes to revel in a liquid world with a maze of soft colors, green and blue mostly, and an intense fiery white. They provide a night time of entertainment as I slide around inside my broken brain.

*   *   *

The tree was magnificent, even leafless in the clear December air. Its massive, roughly rounded, gray structure beckoned the eye on a sensuous path into the air and it took my breath away.

This tree was truly placed and perfectly shaped, something no one could have predicted when it was planted fifty-seven rough years before Joyce and I fell in love with it. Surely, chance and genes conspired to our good fortune. The tree's spreading limbs framed the entire neighborhood and shielded the house from the street and the hot afternoon sun. The way it opened its branches softened the geometric edges of the old, wood structure of our house. Men, it is said, buy cars and women buy houses, and I think there is some truth to that, especially when a tree has been strategically placed. We bought the house for two reasons; one was the tree.

A tree such as our maple insinuates its way into the fabric of life quickly, and before long we depended on it for small but important things. It became a guardian to protect us. It was also a place where squirrels and birds scampered and flitted to the delight of cats. Its leafy coolness in summer made the house comfortable without air conditioning.

You can own a house and shape it to your style and desires with architects, furnishings and paint, but you cannot own a tree in the way you own a house. A tree has a life of its own. After a while, we worried about the way the limbs hung over the roof and thick, dead limbs threatened the upstairs windows.

There was a big, dark hole in the side of the tree, a smooth opening into which squirrels tunneled during the day. In time the tree became a symbol of age and vulnerability. The thick surface roots turned a sidewalk into a 45-degree angle slide that could trip a neighbor. What offered security once turned slowly into a threatening, dark shadow.

About this time I began to think I was lucky I did not own the ground on which the tree stood. It belonged to the county as part of the street right-of-way.

One day I telephoned the county about its tree and how it threatened our house, property and maybe even our lives. The person who answered the phone sent an urban forester to evaluate the situation. To our relief, the county determined that tree removal was too drastic, and a crew arrived to trim the dead, dying and dangerous branches. We were content and secure once again.

Our love for the tree was restored and twenty happy years slid by before a letter arrived from the county. It informed us our tree was one of a hundred selected for removal because it was old and under the electric power lines. Before our house was built about 1917, the land was devoted to agriculture and before that Indians left their footprints everywhere. We took the proposed tree removal in stride, which was unusual because humans accept nothing and alter everything.

Inexplicable delays occurred and the tree was spared another twenty-four months until one December day when two trucks arrived with burly men who wore stiff boots and carried chain saws. The first assault was carried out by lumberjacks skilled in working around power lines. A few days later a second crew arrived to remove the lower portion of the tree, revealing limbs hollow with rot.

A week later the stump removal crew arrived with a huge, evil-looking machine. They proceeded to grind the stump away with noise so loud the crew wore special hearing protectors sticking out from their heads like large plastic earmuffs. The machine roared and whined as it went back and forth over the stump, cutting little bits of wood away with each pass. There was nothing surgical about it. I watched the machine and the burly men but I turned away from the roar of the stump grinder with its heavy, cruel blade because there were tears in my eyes.

Do you want the chips? the foreman asked. They're good for mulch around shrubs. I told him to leave them.

After the workmen left, I looked at the empty place where

the tree had been. All that remained of the tree that was truly placed and perfectly shaped was a four-foot-high mound of tan wood chips cut from its heart. I loaded a cart again and again and spread the maple chips over the garden like human ashes spread over the sea to symbolize the unity of life. It was cold work and the weak December light disappeared before I finished. The work impressed me with the enormity of what had happened in my life with the loss of the tree. An icy vulnerability descended upon me. Before I stopped spreading the chips there were tears in my eyes again.

At a certain age, even cynical old men struggle with the recurring fragility of their own clever bodies. They find the exhilaration of youth vanishes like a giggle on a windy day, replaced with the limp awareness of their own cheap mortality. It is then they discover how difficult it is to part with something truly placed and perfectly shaped.

The spring following the soul-wrenching removal of our old tree was warmed by a brilliant sun and my sadness moderated as I watched the deep green leaves of my day lilies push through the maple chip mulch. I remembered the long, fruitful life of the tree and the way its rich, hard essence returns to the earth as nourishment and provides new promise. Thus does the wealth of a single tree outlive the human memory and become timeless.

It's the middle of the night and I wake up alone with tears pouring down my face and I have a lonely erection.

The old woman was gnomish with a face covered in deep wrinkles. She was dressed in dark clothes. A kerchief over her head was tied under her chin. While her granddaughter shopped, the old woman watched me with growing annoyance as I took money from customers.

It was obvious from her appearance the woman was not of America and, when she finally opened her mouth, broken English with an Italian accent reached my ears. Her message was stern, moralistic, and came from experience in another place and another time. She demanded to know how I could sell herb plants growing wild and free everywhere. She implied I was dishonest in this endeavor. I shrugged. There are more used cars per square foot in the urban fields that surround me than there are weeds of any pedigree. I had no answer for the old woman, but I knew I crossed a moral line in her mind. In another time and place, I would argue the point or attempt to explain the situation.

The old woman in peasant black spoke as directly as Meni and Barbara Checco, my Italian peasant ancestors and men of the earth. We can gain much from those who come from a background of subsistence farming and food gathering from the wild. It teaches us to question many of our modern assumptions.

I spent the first half of my life questioning the large political and philosophical axioms of my times. Now I find comfort and amusement in searching the dirty corners for small, common things holding enlightenment and not anger. I am entering a time of life in which I have begun to quarrel with lingering habits, and the old woman focused my attention on the underclass of horticulture, the plants we call weeds.

Alzheimer's has given me something wonderful. I hear and see things nobody else experiences. They are my truly unique experiences because they occur totally inside my mind and I am unable to define them or describe them. A few of them can be duplicated with my throat, but like a singer, not everybody can sing the notes.

A CHERRY TREE rises from the earth near the southeast corner of the house. Its black branches arch above the red bricks of the patio. The tree is too tall for me to capture all its small, reddish-black fruit in late spring, even from the top of my tallest ladder. For the past few listless years, the fruit on the lower branches has gone unharvested and has been allowed to drop and splatter its dark juice on the bricks and the teak furniture. This cherry tree is in the wrong spot but nobody who lives here thinks about cutting it because its main use has always been as a memorial, not as a tree to bear pleasant, sweet fruit.

The tree is said by neighborhood old-timers to have been a seedling descendant of one of the cherry trees in the orchard covering this land at the turn of the century. It is a small miracle any of those trees remained after the orchard was cleared and roads and houses built. The original cherry tree stood on the property line where my neighbor's bamboo now grows. Its trunk was so large when I pressed my face against its dark rugged bark and hugged it, I could not reach all the way around. After the original tree died, I left its huge trunk standing for many years and thought I might cover it with a vine, but it never happened. I decided finally its living offspring twenty feet away was a better memorial to the fruitful past and we gave the cherry wood from the old trunk to a friend to use in her wood-fired pizza oven.

It is a good thing the cherry tree remained. Not long after we moved into this house my father-in-law, W. K. Doyle, fell in love with the rich fruit it produced. The tree reminded W. K. of his youth. He told us the same story every year about climbing similar trees with his brother, trees that grew around their farm in the foothills of the Blue Ridge Mountains. They stuffed themselves with cherries until they got sick. If W. K. had been raised a druid instead of a Baptist, he could not have had a greater affinity for that cherry tree. He seemed to sense when the fruit was ripe each spring and he showed up ready for a feast when the cherries were at their peak of maturity.

I have a picture of W. K. in the tree. It was taken from the ground looking up at him. He is surrounded by the pointed green cherry leaves with the pronounced ribs on their under-side. His left hand is firmly around a black branch, while his right hand shoves a handful of ripe cherries into his mouth. The cherries already eaten push his belly against his black belt and his yellow polo shirt is wrinkled into long, curved stress lines. Here is a man wreathed with white hair enjoying himself like a kid.

While this picture captures the intensity and joy with which W. K. attacked life, there is another photo of him, taken about the same time, revealing another side of his remarkable person-ality. The photo shows him tipping a straw hat, with an impish grin on his lips and the sparkle of an elf in his eyes. He was the teller of tall tales filled with possums, skunks, frogs and boyish pranks. He could make us howl with yarns about selling straw-berries door to door to scrape up a few pennies, or about his wild rides in a Ford roadster.

He loved to recount his adventures as a young carpenter at work on the Pentagon and of the weekend dances around War-renton. There were occasions when artists and their friends met to celebrate Mardi Gras to the sound of Cajun music in Alexan-dria's Torpedo Factory Art Center in the 1980s, and I caught a glimmer of W. K.'s footwork of a dance-hall past.

All these things I remember and hold dear, but the sharpest image in my memory is of his seventy-fourth birthday, which I celebrated with him during a three-day weekend at a fly fishing school outside Roanoke. When I made reservations for two, I had some misgivings; I thought it would be a delightful week-end and a wonderful birthday present, but would he enjoy it as much as me? He knew nothing about fly fishing, but I'd been dreaming of it for thirty-five years.

My misgivings deepened the week before the trip as I saw his physical condition worsen and his head sag from pain. Three days before the trip W. K. learned he had inoperable cancer. For a man who suffered the pain of heart disease and two heart bypass operations, this news was a real blow. Although he almost passed up the birthday trip, he went. He was not feeling well and the new medicine was making him feel worse.

At breakfast the first morning, W. K. said, I don't feel too good. I don't think I can make the first class. Then he changed his mind. I'll try it for a few hours, he said. After lunch, he was ready to go with the class to the private water where the instruction took place. Little did I suspect the profound experience we were to find in the mountains around Roanoke as still, clear, cold spring water shimmered in a warm afternoon and mayflies mated in pulsing swarms above trout that coursed sensuously through the pond. So much was the area like the misty, green Virginia mountains where W. K. was raised, it must have made him feel as if he'd gone back in time.

On the last day of the class, we had a chance to test how well we had learned our lessons. W. K. stationed himself on the lip of a small dam. I picked a spot about thirty yards upstream near the spring where the creek began.

I looked up from my fishing at the sound of a shout. W. K.'s rod was bent almost double and he danced up and down as he reeled in the first trout, fooling with a bit of wire, fur and feathers. He caught five more big fish in thirty minutes and each time he was as excited as the first. A man near death found something new in life for which to live. Science may not have a cure for something as simple as the common cold or for something as stubborn as cancer or Alzheimer's, but for the maladies of the human soul, fly fishing may be the answer.

W. K. engaged a century in its youth and in its old age, from a time when the nation walked to days when airplanes sparkled in the night sky. In spring I think of W. K. as the cherry tree in my backyard bursts into clouds of white spring flowers and turns green with renewed life. Throughout his seventy-four years, W. K. received great joy from simple pleasures like eating fresh cherries and driving power boats fast over calm water.

When he died in January 1991, our cherry tree took on new meaning. This tree, a refugee from a long-ago cherry orchard, became a symbol of Life, the life contained in a little cherry that spurts sweet juice, and the life of a man who loved the tree and who expressed joy in a vigorous, unclaimed life. Yes, the tree provides a reminder of the past and those who loved it, but there is steady comfort to be found in its passage through the seasons as Nature reminds us that in death life is renewed.

I can feel the memories just below the surface of awakening. It is a difficult place to find words, but in my trance they appear by magic. Small miracles inside my brain.

❋

As my interest in weeds increased and my perception of them altered, I sought understanding instead of destruction. I began to sense nobility in the persistence of weeds. Perhaps they even had something to teach me.

I took a hard look at the dirt in my tiny backyard garden and discovered it had a multifaceted background, if the variety of weeds that sprout there are good indicators. To verify the extent of my weed population, I inventoried it along with two keen-eyed friends of dirt, Dottie Jacobsen and Laura Schneider. Here's what we found: oxalis, pigweed, wild clematis, purslane, chickweed, bermuda grass, ground ivy, *Artemisia vulgaris,* chicory, sumac, wild grape (porcelain vine), crabgrass, bindweed, wild locust, several worts, violets, honeysuckle, plantain, dandelion, poison ivy, wild strawberry, sensitive fern, mimosa, pokeweed, coconut geranium, rose of sharon, spurge, sweet woodruff, mâche and moss. And those were just the plants we could identify.

Pondering this extensive list made me realize weeds are

really just plants I didn't expect to find where they were. This is obvious when you have a population of thyme, rosemary, basil, chives, mâche, dill, lavender, coriander, fennel and parsley sprouting in stony paths and germinating in other uncultivated spots. Less familiar plants sometimes also have fine pedigrees stamped with special attributes of which we are ignorant.

Outside, the air is chipper with large white snowflakes whirling from the sky. I stand in the center of this snowy morning and breathe snow and the unseen air.

In the snow, a quiet afternoon watches without seeing. White flakes fall in windswept whorls and melt on the sidewalk. Without looking up, two men pass hurriedly, disappearing into the night.

Without the Alzheimer's diagnosis, I'd still be a man with dirty hands, weary from interminable days standing on my feet, growing herb plants.

Alzheimer's provided an opportunity for me to give up dirt and search the rocky hillsides of memory for places of hidden freshets still remaining to tell me who I was and where I have been. All around me I am greeted by my failing past, rough places of memories from baby days to dying days, almost all in the same little community.

My years of silence cost the streets a rich memory. Trees sing to me as I walk through the path of memory, while around me the world changes quickly before my hungry eyes. The sin of new bulky high-rise buildings now shades a time of failing memory and nervous decline.

I wake up, tears streaming from my eyes. A strange sound comes from my mouth, a dry half cry for help, half chant of death.

*   *   *

Adrienne Cook, the garden columnist for the *Washington Post,* and I shared weed stories, and soon a package from her appeared in my mailbox. Inside was an extra review copy of a delightful and thorough new book by Pamela Jones called *Just Weeds.* The book sets forth the history, myths and uses of some of our most common weeds.

Jones wrote about many weeds in my garden. Three of the most prolific and persistent uncultivated plants she spotlights are ground ivy, purslane and chickweed. A customer once told me that the scent of crushed ground ivy, a vigorous, evergreen ground cover with small blue flowers, has the power to end headaches. Although it's not one of the claims reported in Jones's book, she does mention ground ivy used to clarify Saxon beer long before hops was used for that purpose. In my early days as a nurseryman, I even potted ground ivy weeds and made hanging baskets of them.

More than 2,000 years ago, East Indians and Persians ate purslane, a green succulent spreading rapidly in my garden and in the gravel paths. Europeans have even gone overboard for this weed and developed cultivated varieties of it to make their salads more tempting. One reason purslane is so persistent is that pulling the stuff actually speeds seed production.

Chickweed has an even more unbelievable past. This small-leaved ground cover spreads so fast over winter in my garden it creates a low, tight, green carpet in a couple of months. Such a common, quick growing plant is bound to have a multitude of medicinal uses, and chickweed has accommodated herbalists for centuries with concoctions to allegedly reduce swelling and cure everything from coughs to hemorrhoids.

I know I can convince myself weeding is a crime against nature, but this isn't the place to try to change human behavior. Weeds, like humans, are full of tenacity, opportunism and patience. When gardeners speak of weeds, however, they mean language filled with bravado and trespass. Instead we should recognize our similarities and welcome weeds as wholesome comrades.

Outside George Mason University, near my house, a middle-aged man hugs a parking meter while he waits for someone.

꧁

THE PHRASE "master gardener" has taken on institutional meaning in recent years as the Agriculture Extension Service has awarded the title to those who take its gardening course. Originally the term meant the likes of Mr. Benjamin King. Few who saw him used the term to define him. They only saw the five-foot-tall old man with long white hair walking along the street. He had a pained gait, the result of arthritis, and it looked as if he were trying to stand upright against a great weight pushing down on his back. It could take him five or ten minutes to walk a hundred yards.

He always carried a cardboard box or two lashed with heavy twine. They swung from his short arms and accentuated the pendulous cadence of his walk. He usually wore the same dirty tee shirt, blue jeans and heavy work boots. On hot, sunny summer days, he covered the top of his head for protection with a brown paper bag folded down to make a cube-shaped hat.

Mr. King was not the embodiment of Warner's credo that "in order to enjoy agriculture, you do not want too much of it." He always wanted more. Why else would he be getting his hands dirty at eighty-seven? But I think he agreed with Warner's notion that it was enough to "hoe while it is spring, and enjoy the best anticipations. It is not much matter if things do not turn out well."

Mr. King scuffed his knuckles and let his own blood to plant trees and create beauty for others. As a boy, he scouted the forests along the Potomac river as a fern picker. Later he helped mold the great gardens at Dumbarton Oaks in Washington, D.C. In his eighties, he was still at it but on a more modest scale, working in a widow's garden down the street.

Through it all he learned the primary lesson Warner thought the private garden taught. "It is not to give the possessor vegetables and fruit (that can be better and cheaper done by the market-gardeners)," Warner wrote, "but to teach him patience and philosophy, and the higher virtues—hope deferred, and expectations blighted, leading directly to resignation, and sometimes to alienation. The garden thus becomes a moral agent, a test of character, as it was in the beginning."

Mr. King's acknowledged reverence for trees revealed his deep philosophic side, nurtured by the time of his life and the long silences imposed on him as a gardener working alone. He often talked about Franklin Roosevelt and he remembered him as the president who began social security.

The presidential stroke of a pen that protected Mr. King's old age also created a dream inside him. He called his dream Birchland, a place much like the biblical Eden, where people lived in harmony among themselves and with nature. Mr. King and I often discussed where Birchland might best be built. He thought a good spot was Kentucky because it had quiet woods and plenty of trees. Such dreams of milk and honey come easily to the very young, who lack both knowledge and experience, and to the very old, worn out by the drudgery of sucking wisdom from their daily labors.

When he died, Mr. King left behind the little house his beloved mother had bequeathed him. He worried over it constantly, but he could do little with it except, like his life, wear it out. My memories of this old gardener are his priceless gift to me. These recollections took on a life of their own in me and grew into appendages as important to my spirit as are my arms and legs to my body. Along with these active remembrances, Benjamin King helped me discover that tears shed over the death of a friend have the power to reinvigorate the poetry and value of life.

For all his appearance as one of the homeless, Mr. King was like a tree himself; he had character and pride that touched others deeply. As a gardener, he had participated in something magnificent, he once remarked. When he died around Christmas 1989, he was not as frail and alone as he seemed. He planted a tree and lived to see it tower above the earth. Birchland did not die with him.

WEEDS THAT BECOME uninvited tenants in gardens remind me of the antisocial side of our nature, the crooked part haunting our moral awareness with mystery, promiscuity and randomness. We fear what we cannot control and do not understand. Surely that describes our modern relationship with weeds, as well as philosophy and politics.

> More than sweet recollections are at stake when memories begin to lose their leaves. Fire scours the brain, disabling mind and body and squeezing what is left of life hanging on a tombstone.

I have often gone to the private places of my life to entertain and enlighten, but this is my last perambulation through memory, a lamentable occurrence made a necessity by events beyond my control.

I have also come to mourn the closing of our Arlington greenhouse after twenty-four years, and to celebrate its consolidation with our spacious Chantilly gardens.

Our small farm has two large heated greenhouses and is near Dulles Airport, only thirty minutes from Arlington. It is nearly five acres, providing us with many advantages over our cramped former quarters in Arlington. We know you will all recognize the value of the large parking lot, and our ability to offer you a larger array of homegrown herb, vegetable and ornamental plants. This new location provides us an opportunity to bring you expert speakers, both local and national, to provide information to make your gardening easier and more successful.

For many years, you and I listened to each other and gained from the conversation. It was not just friendly banter and it made herb and vegetable gardens flourish. In the process we became friends, and it is as a friend that Ol' Peeps appears now to acknowledge the wonder of this relationship that began for some of you a quarter century ago.

From the first Saturday we sold plants from a front yard card table, our goal has been to offer the highest quality and the largest selection of varieties. From the beginning we were different. Unlike many large nurseries, we grew the plants we sold. We never hesitated to discard plants not meeting our standards and we developed new ways to assure quality and value. Along the way we developed many new herb varieties and we continue to play with the gene pool at our nursery, and around the United States looking for new herbs to brighten your gardens.

The concepts guiding us from the beginning are old-fashioned garden homilies remembered from childhood; it was worth preserving them twenty-five years ago and it is worth keeping them today. I noticed early that this approach created a deep and complex relationship between buyer and seller, and it could be very personal. We got used to that and liked it very much, and we became friends with you in spite of the fact money was involved.

Before long Ol' Peeps got into the act. The stylized moniker that characterized him came from a column written for a little weekly paper in Delaware. The name "Peeps" was used to emphasize the disreputable wink the ol' boy had. Visually Peeps was the least inviting gent imaginable, even a bit evil, but the absurd winking head made the ol' boy laugh. We needed Peeps desperately that spring to help fill an empty place in the catalog that looked embarrassing without words because we had no more garden talk. After his introduction, he quickly became a quirky centerpiece of the catalog.

My relationship with you prospered and more greenhouses popped up in our backyard, and then, with a nudge from the county, we decided to consolidate everything into one building. It was a single, bright greenhouse with plenty of room and it covered most of our backyard. It was a place in which nothing was hidden; the finished plants for sale were on one side of the building and the growing plants were on the other. It fit our idea of openness and trust perfectly.

Everything went along well until one day last spring when an accumulation of small events rang a bell and I told my family doctor I was having trouble identifying by name and character-istics some of the plants I had known intimately for many years. My memory loss began in a small way, I realized in hindsight, at least a year earlier, and it was complicating my life, to say the least.

Joyce and I thought the culprit was stress and worry and the long, hard days. During a routine physical, I told my family doc-tor of my memory loss. He immediately referred me to a spe-cialist at Georgetown University Hospital. I met with him in early March and a schedule of tests began. The testing was slow but it was finished the end of May. I was told I had Alzheimer's, a destructive neurological disease with no cure.

The type of Alzheimer's I have is rare, striking patients between thirty and sixty. I am fifty-seven. The tests indicated I had severely impaired short-term memory and poor episodic memory. It was a pattern, the report of the neuropsychological evaluation concluded, that was "entirely consistent with early stage Alzheimer's Dementia."

Although the disease has been known for nearly a hundred years, its secrets have been revealed slowly and only recently. Not enough is known today of Alzheimer's to stop or satisfactorily control its evil destruction of the brain. Fortunately, the horizon is bright with possibilities to control and even reverse the disease.

I hoped to follow my grandmother DeBaggio's long life. I wanted to beat her 104 years. Without the intervention of a medical miracle to reverse the Alzheimer's, it is more likely I will follow my parents and repeat their early deaths.

There are few things in life as tasty as basil, as worthwhile to have in the garden as rosemary, and as sweet as the aroma of lavender, but even they need to be renewed periodically and it is that process on which Francesco, Joyce and the men and women who work with us have now embarked. Although I must bow out in time, I intend to hang around as long as I can and work as hard as I ever have to grow the finest plants possible. I may not be as visible in the greenhouse in the days to come but I will be there in person frequently and in spirit forever.

You have been a large part of my life and when I was not producing plants for you, I was thinking about you. You have been my lifeline for the last twenty-five years. I am going to miss you.

I never thought I would have to write words so personal and sad they opened the secret places in my heart. Tears fill my eyes as I write these final words. This is not the end but the beginning of a new adventure, different from all others, uncharted, mysterious and frightening. It is a journey we all take some time in our life, and it is the final thing we do.

*   *   *

Yesterday during my morning walk I saw a man riding a bike through busy rush hour traffic. The cyclist sat
back on the seat, relaxing without holding the handlebars.

The plants we cultivate so carefully contain our dreams and our
garden's future. Weeds are plants that threaten to interfere with
those dreams. It is our nature to destroy what we perceive as a
threat to our future, so we pull the weeds and toss them on the
compost pile. Weeds deserve better; they are often someone
else's cultivated plants.

Unexpected plants from self-sown seeds form a basic record
of the horticultural past. They are promiscuous, with an open
but benevolent, opportunistic morality of their own. They create
an underground living memory colored with struggle, hardship
and unhappiness. These are like the unkind memories humans
sometimes try to forget.

Weeds, like those rough spots in our own past, are not easily
forgotten and continually return to haunt us, and that may be
the key to our complex relationship with these freelance plants
sprouting wherever there are quiet, empty spaces.

Memory is the most intimate of the muses, particular
to each individual. Its loss empties the mind and leaves
one forever a cripple and soon a corpse.

The cherry tree, only a sapling when it was first ours, is now
a rough, dark, dead obelisk, a trunk slowly deteriorating on the
spot from which it sprang many years ago. It is accidentally
dead from our own hands when we cut large, important roots
under the yellow clay to make room for the two fish pools
backed up to the house today.

On the side of the house next to the bamboo, Joyce has turned
her talents to creating a flower garden between the tall bay trees

and the sidewalk over which customers formerly saw bench after steel bench of plants sunning themselves against our house. The walk begins at the parking lot and ends at the greenhouse, now a dishonored figure full of memories and dust and decaying plants. It is a place like a cave with hidden wealth somewhere under the steel benches, now full of luxuriant weeds. It is a place that waits for spring thrushes and other birds. The greenhouse is a memorial now to a man still alive but no longer all there.

I shut my eyes, and instead of darkness, I am treated to a liquid world full of mazes and soft colors. There is a subtle pulsing in the lights as they swim before me. When I fall asleep, I know the light show will be waiting tomorrow.

I do not know when or how I will die. Pick a day. Use the lottery. I think little of death; my body reminds me of it with every breath. My death is acknowledged all around me. It was in me from birth and only now do I recognize its structure.

It is likely to be a long struggle, full of grief, torment, misunderstanding and abiding sorrow all around me. That is a typical death by Alzheimer's. Every death is different, it is often said.

I find these thoughts difficult to understand because today I am loaded with energy, and the ideas, blocked for many days, have shown plentifully in their own secret ways. Right now I feel I will not tinkle away for sometime.

It is even possible you will not know I am dead at all. One day I will float away on a cloud and a breeze, leaving the solid and the sunlight for a new mortality as quick as running water.

I see an end sometime, not actually a vision of it, but perhaps the way a novelist might see it. When I picture my death, it is magical. What a silly idea. It reveals how far from a real death I am. I will not go silently from this world.

*   *   *

I am writing my life while crouched on curb stones, obedient to the Muse.

I have little experience with death. Luck, I suspect. I watched my silent mother for several days while a sharp cold ruled Eldora, Iowa. I watched her waste away slowly, a chip of ice for sustenance, until there was nothing more, no more reason to live, nothing left.

Joyce's father's death was not so surprising. He cheated his death for years and kept recovering remarkably from an angry heart, until there was no place to hide. My mother-in-law died almost the way she lived, a secret anger governed by dreams and disappointments, until she became so thin she disappeared.

Now my term is in sight. Will it be five, ten, fifteen years? The doctor will not speculate and neither will I. If I am correct and die within the year I pick, it will prove nothing.

Every day I search for clues offering hints of the future. What I see today is vocabulary diminishing and letters within words appropriating their own language, where the letter "P" replaces "B", or a "T" for a "D", blurring my ability to write clearly. I am stumbling, and as my brain continues to fail I will no longer understand the structure of words. I may continue to believe in words for periods of time, but in a way not taught in school. I am slowing reverting to early childhood. What wonders may be there I don't expect to report. I can live without speaking but what happens without understanding?

This afternoon my brain sent me a message in the usual way. In the silence of my workroom, the image walked into my brain from wherever they are sent. I have relied on such messages for years as a writer and I do not doubt them nor do I try to understand their genesis. In this case I was given a chance to walk down the hall to my workroom. I gently opened the door, normally so difficult to open it speaks to me. There is a man sitting at my desk. He has turned on all the flourescent tubes to brightly illuminate the work area, which as usual is piled with scraps of paper with notes jotted on them.

I wondered who was sitting at my desk because I had not heard anyone come into the house this afternoon. From where I am standing by the door, it appears the man sitting in my chair has reached to write something on a piece of white paper with the pen he holds in his right hand. I walk over to the figure and look closely at the lifeless body. On the desk is a slim paperback book, *Malone Dies,* a work by Samuel Beckett. I notice the dead man has an uncanny resemblance to me. He is sitting where I was last night, reading this book. It seems the man at the desk died an illuminated death with a favorite book.

Fish fight in a languid pool for tiny morsels of food on
a foggy morning dripping with memory

In the desert of concrete and asphalt that blossoms with used-car lots around me, I admire the fecundity of loose gravel and Virginia clay, but I know it is the exception and not the rule. I never lose my admiration for the little rosemary seedlings that push up through the gravel paths in the garden but I am equally astounded by the chickweed covering the garden during winter.

In the garden, we bestow accolades on those plants least adaptable whose lives depend most on us, and treat as trash the plants most adapted to our climate and soil.

So barren is my life now that you will find me looking
at the world through a furtive slat in the bathroom shade
like a spy in a tree.

As I grow older with Alzheimer's, I become more open. Last weekend was the perfect example. Home Box Office (HBO) bought a small part of the last of my life and I am connected to the entertainment company through two men, Dan Collison and Tom Jennings. They are freelancers, whose job it is for a few days every three or four months to follow me around with cameras in their eyes to catch the reality of a man dying such a slow death nobody recognizes it. Eventually, their visits will be put together for a special documentary on Alzheimer's. It is more fun than struggle.

On their most recent visit, we started out from my house and drove in separate cars to Dr. Blanchfield's office at Seven Corners. While we waited I caught occasional flashes of the doctor working in her suite of offices behind the waiting room. Piles of magazines covered tables in the waiting room, but none of them tickled me. I sat in silence, watching the little waterfalls on the other side of the room chattering away.

It wasn't long before the doctor was ready and Dan and Tom took their positions, lenses to their eyes, one inside the office, the other just outside the door. The doctor and I talked of things we always talk about, my Alzheimer's and how the medicines are working. We decided to make a slight change in one of the two medications I take, reducing the dose of Exelon. The medicines have no curative power, one of the great drawbacks of the prescriptions available as the year 2000 ended. She gave me several tests, as she does each visit. The tests examine memory. One tests my memory of some colored balls. Another examines my ability to reproduce a drawing.

After the doctor learned there were few events to talk about, I went to the waiting room to cool my heels while Dan and Tom spent a good amount of time with the doctor. They call it their "debriefing." When it is over, she is out of the building before us. She doesn't have regular office hours on Fridays.

For this visit in early October, I have put together a series of stops at shops I frequent. This gives the HBO tramps a chance to get footage of me in the real world instead of having me stare into a camera while they whip me with questions.

At Arrow Wine, the first stop, I selected a couple of bottles.

Then we headed for Angler's Lie where we got advice on tackle to fish Mossy Creek, a little trout stream two hours' drive in the foothills of the Blue Ridge Mountains. Francesco and I planned to fish Monday. After we finished at the fly shop we headed for lunch at the Greek Taverna.

On the way back from lunch, Dan and Tom drove their rental car alongside me and got in front of me. I realized Dan was filming me through the back window of their car. After a while, they motioned me to pull over. Dan wanted to film me driving while he leaned out the front passenger side window. And so began one of the most peculiar car rides I have ever encountered.

As I drove along nonchalantly, Dan hung far out his car window while Tom drove. With the camera in his eye, he shot film of me driving from every conceivable angle, including a long stretch where their car was only halfway in the right lane. Before the episode was over there was a long slow line of cars behind us. I was relieved when we got back to the Angler's Lie to pick up our tackle and have another indoctrination on the ways to catch trout on Mossy Creek.

The afternoon was devoted to a lengthy interview in my workroom and a walk down the street, after which we went to Alexandria to Joyce's studio at the Torpedo Factory Art Center. Joyce is not happy about strangers probing her life, and she is permitting it only because we both agree there may be some value to others in telling our story. Tom and Dan are trying to film enough footage to tell our story, as sad and happy as it is, and they are quietly tenacious. Take Tom and Dan from their cameras and they are just ordinary guys who have seen a lot.

There are days now when the imaginative shadow that has followed me since childhood appears to be a threatening apparition.

*   *   *

Tom Jennings went back to New York, leaving Dan to dog Francesco and me on our Monday fishing adventure, the first of the year for the two of us although trees were shedding leaves already. For Dan this must have been in the dregs of the story, but he was chipper when he arrived at the farm, after waking a little earlier than usual.

To watch an angler on Mossy Creek is to see patience and careful craft. The stream at its widest is probably not more than fifteen feet. It meanders through three miles of fallow ground. On a large part of this old farmland, weeds six feet high grow right up to the edge of the water, making fishing difficult. In summer and fall, anglers are likely to head upstream from the little parking area above the creek to avoid the tall grass. My reason to go was not to fish as much as it was to say a long good-bye to a place that has meant much to me off and on for many years.

There were many layers of Mossy Creek memory still stored in my brain, and as I drove the car much of it bubbled up. It was a place of frequent failure, a character that mirrored me, and a place of stillness and hope. In a lonely place like Mossy Creek you confront failure and see fine things come from it, especially the desire to push ahead no matter the barriers.

Francesco and I got our gear on and went our separate ways, as is usual. Dan stayed with Francesco and I disappeared, headed three miles away for the cold beginnings where the springs begin. It was here I wanted to say good-bye to a place rich in memory, not for an angler, but as a place of contemplation. It is a spot where I learned the importance of failure, and its inevitability.

It was at Mossy Creek many years ago on a frigid overcast winter day I devoted myself to emptiness and discovered its charm and necessity. It was like taking a bath with your skin removed. All the parts were spread out to see in their fine shapes.

It was here understanding, as singular and robust as a dust mote, began to take place inside me.

It was here I imagined the stalactites that inhabit the deep caves nurturing the cold waters flowing steadily in silence.

It was here I learned how to peel back layers of memory left in times unprepared for tomorrow.

I LOOKED UP from where I sat in the Mossy Creek weeds of long ago and saw a car slip into the narrow little parking area next to mine. A teenager got out while his mom stayed behind the wheel of the car. It was late on a winter afternoon.

The boy got his equipment quickly and headed off upstream. I knew the place to stop first, an area where the stream passes through a deeply cut bank where you can see the large fish on the bottom waiting for the sun to drop and the bugs to come out on the water.

Mom opened her book and began to read in the failing light, waiting for the moment when darkness brought her son back with a smile on his face and a feeling of self-fulfillment.

ALL INTERVIEWERS HAVE their own style; some are dogged, others lackadaisical and plodding. No matter the style, Joyce does not like the process. She is nervous and does not want to get caught exposing her self. This has brought about a distinct tension between Joyce and Dan and Tom. The idea of spilling the beans is anathema to Joyce, but to the storytellers it is the gold mine of truth. Trying to bring them together has been a trial for me. I don't know how it will turn out. I just talked to Dan and he is thinking about taking us to dinner when he is here next time. I don't think the method is what is making Joyce hold back. The release of private memory keeps Joyce clammed up.

In unguarded moments, I am robbed of memories every day, severing me from my life.

The interviews conducted by Dan and Tom, the HBO documentary makers, are like the debriefing of an astronaut just returned from an unknown planet. Actually my brain is a strange place of wonder and tears, more mysterious than outer space and much closer. But sometimes I am as lonely and bewildered as a space cadet, shivering with fear and death. Water and dreams come together on the good days. The top spins without a wobble.

On an orange towel, dark with the shape of a cat, a clock chimes in deep blue color. When days like this come, I am full and alone. I wait for the fish to splash me.

❦

LIVING NEXT TO a used-car lot is full of uncertainties and surprises. Joyce and I grew up surrounded by trees and colorful, crunchy, fall leaves. Living in a house with a pristine view of parked automobiles gave us a new way to see the world, and a number of surprises.

At night, after the sales people leave for the day, car hounds inspect cars glowing under the bright lights high above on slender steel. When we were in a kindly mood, the lights created a lonely, romantic atmosphere.

Between us and the bright used-car lot is a large area where cars are parked bumper to bumper. There was a lot of foot traffic here as well, especially late at night. Watching the silent lot through a darkened upstairs window was major entertainment for a family without a television.

One morning I awoke early and took a peep out the bathroom window that looks down on the used cars. Morning activity started early with cars brought in every day, but today there was something different. Several men were inspecting the autos. It was not unusual to see people looking under hoods at engines. On this morning there was a cacophony of sound from hoods closing.

It took a while before I translated the usual from the unusual. Finally I realized two men were removing the batteries from each car in the lot. They left each battery beside the front wheel of the car. They were bold and unaware anyone was watching their early thievery. It took a while for me to realize a major battery theft was under way. It wasn't long before police cars came silently from all directions in response to my call.

When theft protection devices first became available there were screaming cars day and night from the used-car lot, but they were usually shut off quickly. One night, long after everybody had left, a vehicle began singing. By eleven P.M. Joyce, Francesco and I had all the auto serenading we could stand, and I went over to see which car was the out-of-tune baritone. I found it and looked around, but I couldn't find any way to turn it off. We stuffed our ears with cotton and tried to sleep that night.

At daybreak the car still sang, but the tune was sliding into a new, quieter sound. Several police officers noticed the commotion when they drove by, but they could do little. Before long the car's battery gave out and there was welcome quiet at last.

There was some car theft from the lot. The most unusual occurred one summer night. You'd think, with the windows open to cool the house, we could hear a car being stolen in the middle of the night next door, but we didn't hear the car plow over the four-foot-high brick wall and drive away with a load of teenagers. The car turned up about four miles away soon after daybreak, with an empty gas tank.

In this quasi-urbane place, almost anything can happen. Yesterday a county fire engine was parked at the supermarket. Even firemen need to eat.

While I worked putting up small, narrow greenhouses and tried to build a mailing list of families eager to grow their own food, I worked for two art supply stores owned by Frank Buckly. I worked for him in Arlington earlier after Joyce and I married.

Kostos was a well-known picture frame shop in Georgetown and Frank had bought it while I skipped from Indiana and Delaware searching for a berth in journalism. Georgetown is a clubby area of expensive townhouses, brick sidewalks and small specialty shops. It was a place with a littered past and precious space to park cars on the narrow one-way congested streets.

Frank's stores, in Georgetown and Arlington, sold art supplies, but much of the business was picture framing. The group working the Georgetown store when I arrived had been together several years and they distrusted me as a newcomer. Their greatest fear was my work earlier in Arlington for Frank. I had his trust. They had good reason to be wary.

Frank was suspicious of what was going on in Kostos. There were usually two large, active dogs present in the narrow little shop. After a few months, all the former employees left for other jobs, and we had a slim staff with the picture framing area now in the basement of the store. I asked Frank in the spring if I could sell plants I grew in the little greenhouse at home, and he encouraged me, knowing I would eventually leave again to grow herbs and vegetables.

I was close to Frank in those days but the relationship was

not the way it was earlier. He went through a divorce and that might have chipped something from a secret place. His great dream then was to live in Maine and one winter he moved there and left me in charge of his business. We got occasional photographs showing the high snow banks. Frank complained about having to shovel snow and when he came back in the spring he was soured on Maine.

The time came quietly for me to leave, before Frank was ready. I left and stuck to my backyard business full-time. Before long Frank sold the Georgetown building and then he shut the Arlington facility. I was sad to see his dream dribble away. We talked on the phone once or twice about old times, and new.

He started drinking again, something he knew he could not handle. I got a call from him in the night darkness; he was in Fairfax County Jail. He had drunk too much and was picked up, incoherent and unsteady on a sidewalk. I got him out of jail the next day and took him home. Later he moved to California, and I lost contact with him.

The night sky was smooth and crystal clear. Airplanes floated through the darkness, blinking lights while trick-or-treat children ran through the sidewalk night in costumes revealing the icon of my death.

❋

THE GREENHOUSE SPREADING across most of the backyard was a bustling place two years ago, with customers pushing their way in to buy plants. Now it is silent in the November cold, empty of human habitation. A scattering of potted rosemary plants and a few other herbs are all that remain. It should be empty, awaiting removal, and Joyce and I complain it is there.

I cannot part with this old greenhouse, too big now for what little use a backyard gardener needs. It may be empty of plants, but for me it holds precious memories of my last twenty-five years, a happy, sometimes lonely period in which I made a small mark in the world where plants and herbs are discussed.

I am afraid when this large reminder of my past in the backyard is removed, I will lose all the precious memories sequestered there and I will be naked and alone. I am afraid of forgetting who I am. This place made me as much as did my parents. I invented myself in this greenhouse and in others less grand. For me this place has a memory thick with emotion and ghosts.

The old greenhouse is a repository of much memory. In itself it is also a personal memorial of my time on earth. If I were separated from it, I worry I might lose the memories it holds. A once inhabited place, empty and vulnerable with age, remains a repository of memory outside the body, and as Alzheimer's presses upon me, squeezing memory from my present, I must rely on other repositories for what memory I can muster.

Every day I enter the greenhouse as if it were a church. I do not genuflect as I might have as a young child. I sprinkle water on the plants in their pots to keep alive the living. I look around this arching building filling the backyard and my life, and I scream until I am hoarse and the tears no longer come. This is the solitary place where I go to bark and loosen the tension of living with Alzheimer's.

The woman with smoky skin huddles against the cold wind as the sun comes up on a Tuesday morning.

It was a long time between visits to the National Arboretum in Washington, D.C. It is a large area of rolling land, a natural place to dream. The special little space set aside for those devoted to herbs has special meaning for me.

In the days when I made frequent trips, the Arboretum meant herbs and Holly Shimazu, a friend and herb aficionado who later became better known to the rest of America on television. These happy, new days with herbs and dirt brought me great happiness and friendship. I was lucky to be in the right place at the right time: the Arboretum, the Herb Society, and in gardens of herbs.

As Francesco drove me to the Arboretum that day, his first look at the place he had heard so much about, I tried to dig into my memories of the place. There was a speaking engagement with Susan Belsinger I remember without much detail. There were annual spring plant sales bringing income to me as a grower. I remembered the open ground Holly prepared for the plants, a few of which I provided. Most of the plants were small and after planting there wasn't much show for several years. I remember a few visits to take cuttings and swap plants and then it seems everything disappeared. There was little more left in my jittery brain.

What Francesco and I found at the Arboretum was new to us both. His eyes were bright and excited; mine were weary, covered in a mental mist. I remembered almost nothing and Francesco pointed out for me some of the plants I had named during a time when I tried my hand at breeding herbs.

The Arboretum was a place for me to look for evidence I was once in this world. In another way, I saw it as a cemetery of my dreams. Francesco was kind and curious and I explored dirt and herbs with him, as if for the first time. It was a day he remembered more than I did.

This day's adventure was part of the tour of unexpected familiar haunts. I visited many of these places for what I envisioned as the last time. I was saying good-bye to the plants at the Arboretum and to the few memories of the place I still had. It was good to see the words that represented my breeding work on new plants. There were names like Tucker's Early Purple, W. K. Doyle, Joyce DeBaggio and more I no longer remember.

After we left the Arboretum I felt I returned to a grave site and walked over a private family cemetery full of pieces of my life. It was a place that was familiar and at the same time full of uncertainty.

It was here on this lovely day at the end of October I took another look at my life. I found myself wondering whether any of this was true. I was uncertain I was ever here before, but I saw the familiar tombstones, touched them with eyes and hands. The visit, whether to a cemetery or a field of memory, did not bring happiness or real understanding.

The day told a story, but not the one I hoped to read. There were occasional bright lights and laughter. It was more somber than I expected and at the same time it was a walk through a garden full of my life; I just wasn't all there anymore.

The chaos of my mind is like a drunkard in a story, tipsy and wandering.

While I was walking this morning, a man passed me on the way to work. I got a whiff of his cologne and it brought back stale memories of my father fifty years ago, and I barked in that peculiar lonely, scared way of Alzheimer's, a frightening scream of hurt and loss, full of secrets. The death of my parents many years ago comes back to haunt me now in ways it never has. When you carry death inside your body, you are no longer the person you once were, although the world does not see how you have changed. You see the world differently with every breath.

The house on Ivy Street is choked with waiting death.

I carry a watering can through Joyce's new flower garden. It is between the house and the neighbor's tall, whispering bamboo that provides unwanted shade. I stop in midstride, unable to remember why I was carrying the watering can. I feel helpless and angry and I scream as I throw the watering can to the ground.

I go inside to hide and cry with frustration. I find an empty house and let go an angry bark directed at the loneliness in which I live and the helplessness of having within me a dying brain.

There are some rare days when I think I could spend hours staring into empty space without a single thought to entertain me.

I remember years ago, before the garden was planted, there was rough, untamed grass to entertain our imagination. After all the green sod was peeled away, yellow clay was everywhere. Then the greenhouses came and it was hard to find a memory of how the backyard looked when I first saw it, before I dreamed myself into a new world.

I created something surprising and startling in the backyard. The earth remains shaped as it was, but there are new visions arriving every day that I will not see. It is too late for me to enter into a new realm. Earth is eternal, memory is fleeting.

The body is only memory's host. Memory is life, the beginning to the end. Without memory there is nothing but the wind burning your face, and the sun.

Last night for Francesco's birthday we scurried to see Cirque du Soleil inside a cold November tent next to a shopping center with cop cars flashing blue and streets burning with police flares. The night and the performance were full of magic lights moving through bodies floating to the roof. It was casual surrealism with a French sensibility. Fading images, in and out of focus, left me breathless.

During intermission Joyce turned to me and said, pointing to my right, "There's Clay." We walked over to see him and the woman who unofficially nurses him. He is an emaciated man with a bony head and hollow cheeks, a vision of the death still alive.

Clay suffers from AIDS, contracted years ago. He still goes to his studio at the Torpedo Factory Art Center in Alexandria, where busybodies shun him and try to lock his studio away from him. Weak, unsteady at times, Clay still works magic in his life and with the creativity he still possesses in his artistic hands.

All around I see the dead and dying, hidden, emaciated bodies chewed up by life until the earth beckons. Yet Clay, devilishly weak at times, goes on breathing new life for others while he dies. (Clay died during the writing of this book. His work as an artist was memorialized in an obituary in the *Washington Post*.)

Every spring I am transported by the wonder of delicate little stems pushing their way into the spring sunlight.

I look in the mirror and see a young man surrounded by tears and hope.

In EARLIER YEARS, before the feline leukemia scare, our neighborhood was full of wandering cats, but there has never been the equal of Sam, a cat once described as all head and balls. He was brought to the neighborhood one summer by the family across the street and we were never the same.

Sam looked like a raccoon, all fur, head and feet. His ears were small, as were his eyes, but his jaw was enormous. We got to know him as a baby. He was always looking for food and he did not stay small. He had a voracious appetite, perhaps because his "owners" across the street never fed him. Our yard was a good hunting ground if the number of squirrel carcasses we found were a gauge. He liked squirrel meat best and when he was finished there was little left, usually a head and maybe some fur.

A friendlier cat I have yet to meet. He'd jump into my lap quickly without an invitation. Even customers who came to our backyard greenhouse for plants fell in love with him. He was gentle enough to let people drape him around their necks.

Sam was everywhere, a free spirit, in a time just discovering feline leukemia. Through the tears of time I can see this big cat shaking with the chills of this deadly disease with nowhere to go for warmth but a hole in the summer ground. Helpless to help the cat, I watched him shiver in the sun one day.

I was so emotionally broken by Sam's illness I could not go to the vet with Joyce and hear the death sentence. Animals become part of you and your family if you let them, part of a living world full of grass, trees, water and wonder.

Joyce remembers how weak Sam was, yet in her arms while the vet watched silently the cat purred in the heavy, happy way the animal owned. The vet, so young and inexperienced in such matters, had trouble sticking the poisoned syringe and took the cat to another room and shaved some of the hair away, frightening the cat further. When he returned, he gave Joyce the cat and Sam continued to purr. While she held the cat, the doctor plunged the deadly syringe into Sam, but instead of killing the sick animal immediately, life lingered a moment or two more before the cat died in Joyce's arms. Joyce lost her father later that year, and then our two indoor cats.

As I try to remember those honeyed days with Sam, I cannot remember much of what happened, but the emotion of those events came flooding back as I typed this sentence and my eyes became so liquid I saw nothing but a blur and I began honking emotionally deep from inside my throat.

*   *   *

This morning I watched my cat Sabina sniff memories from the cold air coming through the kitchen window. She has not been outdoors in years, living inside our cocoon, sharing a view of the outside and an occasional sniff of cold air.

The year Joyce lost her father to cancer two of our cats, Prince and Princess, also died. They were with us through anguish and laughter for fifteen years. From that first day when they hid so well from us we thought they had escaped from a locked house, they brought us new ways of looking at the world. By looking at animals, wild or tamed, and studying their movements and methods we learn about them, but we also discover things about ourselves. These are important things but not large. The longer I carry Alzheimer's, the more I find myself seeking memories, even little shards to lick. It is a vain attempt to remember who I was and who was scattered around me.

I have lived with many cats and their deaths always brought me private choking and tears. There are so many differences between cats and humans, it seems unlikely there could be communication, but there is. The cats use their bodies and sounds to teach us ways to understand them and at the same time we communicate with them and share some of our ways. These are small things, little bits of understanding, and it is the kind of thing I understand on my clumsy way to death.

These are small things in a global sense, but for those emotionally involved they are important. The death of a cat or a dog is as serious to those who lived with it as a human death. It is a trembling, emotional time. That was the way it was when Prince and Princess died but it was also a time full of joy because two new, young cats we named Una and Sabina came into our lives.

*   *   *

Laundry drying on lines beside stationary houses while Francesco and I move fast but notice no movement as the car in which I ride zips along a macadam highway. We whiz by boarded-up buildings in sad, rural Delaware.

A CINDER BLOCK sits beneath where the patio rises six to eight inches above the sidewalk. At first the narrow, rough cinder block appears normal but there is a small dark brown bird stuck in the open space interior of the cinder block. The bird is lifeless but I didn't notice it there earlier today, leading me to believe the peculiar death took place this afternoon. I pull gently on the bird's head but the body does not move. It appears as if the bird backed into the chamber of the cinder block, but there are a few inches between the block and the patio.

A few inches away from where the limp head of the bird extends from the cinder block is a small, loose pile of smooth, light feathers that match the color of the bird. The scene suggests there was some kind of struggle after the bird caught itself. The crime scene is full of ambiguity.

There is no poetry here, only a simple lonely death sometime during election day, Tuesday, November 7, 2000.

The splashing sounds of the water in the nearby fish ponds suddenly fill my ears, washing away this still life of death.

Ducks dance through a honking Delaware sky in long sweeping lines, following their destiny through a wandering sky on a chilly November morning.

Early morning, before the sun owns the sky, is the best time of the day for me and my cats; our memories tremble with the excitement of a new day. It is the time when the world is still, a time when my brain is clearest. When I am lucky, memories present themselves and I begin my day knowing who I am, where I have been, and whether I will have luck prospecting for words. My cats, Sabina and Una, by their presence alone, help me remember who I am when I can't.

The cats have not been outdoors in years, living with us and the various views of the world from windows around the house. Una is overweight and lost her capacity to run and jump, things Sabina is happy to remind her of throughout the day.

I recognized their ability to remember soon after the cats were given to us. The first time Joyce and I drove them to the vet they were unhappy, screaming in their little carry cages. After the first time, just the sight of the carry cage made them disappear. As far as they knew, getting into the cage meant one thing—a visit to the vet, and they wanted none of it.

Of our cats, Sabina is always the first to remind me she is hungry. She guides me from my bedroom door down the winding, painted wood staircase to the first floor of the house. She hurries ahead of me and stops to make sure I am behind her at the entrance to the kitchen. Once in the kitchen she camps in front of the cabinet in which her cat food cans are kept. The minute I come into the room, she begins to serenade me with loud screams. A deaf cat like Sabina has one sound, loud and demanding. I feed her and Una, and head back upstairs to shave and shower.

When I return to the kitchen fifteen minutes later, the cats have eaten. Sabina is spread out at the base of the black refrigerator and begins talking to me in our secret language. She wants to play now and a long black string does the job. When I am tired of playing (she never wearies but I do), it is time for her to have a look at the world as it comes out of darkness. I place a chair near the kitchen sink, and she quickly leaps to the chair and then bounds to the counter in front of the window. She begins to sniff everywhere, especially where my gloves wave to her from a small wicker basket.

While she examines what happened on the counter since she was there last, I open the window. A cool breeze fills the kitchen and Sabina takes her place on the windowsill, stretched out so her entire body fills the space. From this perch she begins sniffing memories and occurrences from the outdoor air as it comes through the window and into the kitchen. She cannot hear the birds but she is excited by their presence in the branches that press against the house. I do not know whether she retains the memory of the day the vet cleaned her teeth and he decided to remove a tooth without informing us. She was overdosed by the vet and nearly died. It is something burned into my memory, and I expect it resides in an angry, private spot in Sabina's memory, too. The overdose left Sabina deaf.

Our second cat, Una, is quite different from loud, often raucous Sabina, but she too is full of vivid memories that haunt her. She came into our life from a waiter we met in a restaurant. He came across a pregnant feral cat, and kept track of it. When the cat gave birth during a thunderstorm in a water-filled basement of an apartment house, he found the kittens nearly drowned. It was such a horrid incident it left a stigma of fear in Una's brain. She is so sensitive that long before dark thunderclouds appear in the sky, she is visually aware of the coming storm and takes refuge in our basement. This dark damp place must have some of the characteristics of the place where she was born. We know the storm is over when she reappears. Her sensitized memory works more accurately than the weather report.

White houses made from old wreckage stand at rural attention. Plowed farm ground surrounds a blown-out house that once held dreams and tears. There is an emptiness along these Delaware roads, and angry memories unconnected to this time and place. Where once there was life, the ground is hunkered in woodlots. As we hurry along these empty roads of sorrow, the rest of the world, stuck in traffic, natters about politics.

*   *   *

Brightly colored leaves fall in a frenzy as winter approaches.
Wind rustles along the bare street catching litter and whipping
it into the air where it skips along out of control. Now is the season time ends and begins again, a clock ticking while generations ask fresh questions. Through all the changes and thick
clouds, the sun eventually burns the morning mist, revealing a
new day washed clean of memory.

I am a voice from an early grave.

Moments of stillness and emptiness inhabit me often now. I stare
into space devoid of thought, blank as a fresh piece of paper. I
am still, inside and out, breathing softly and unresponsively,
while the world spins around me. In this quiet time, I am
unaware of living or dying. I am whole and empty. I see movement without response. I am alive but lost.

The dark night streets bang with urgent honking. The heavy
fire engines come alive with flashing lights and shivering
pyrotechnics. They disappear as quickly as they came, running
red lights at the congested intersection. Weekend stillness settles
in the wake of the noise, impatience, and heightened fear.

The thick black night outside the kitchen window moves
slowly like a river flowing past a sleeping campground. The air
is thick with the blur of branches mimicking dancing couples
who float outside the kitchen windows.

We create holidays such as Christmas to satisfy the part of us
that craves excitement and escape from reality. After many such
holidays, the enthusiasm dims and diversion is less successful.
The words "Merry Christmas" take on a tinny sound, an echo of
the hollowness that precedes insincerity.

Later in life one realizes the holiday is actually a symbol to honor every day in which the love of two people for each other grows deeper and their understanding of each other and the earth becomes greater. From this knowledge comes satisfaction and quiet, sustained joy.

It may be impossible to restore meaning to the phrase "Merry Christmas." Instead of repeating the hollow greeting of these two commercialized words, I wish you love, affection, tenderness and compassion all the days of our life together.

> At night I pull the covers up to my chin and listen to the wind. I roll over and try to sleep but the lights are so bright within my shut eyes that sleep eludes me. With time the lights dim and darkness descends inside my head and I sleep while my brain rots in the humble places.

JOYCE'S FATHER LAY thin and sallow on a narrow daybed. Little sun reached his whiskered face and pale smile, while the wind shivered the fallen leaves into dry, colorful queues, all the way from the low-slung house down through the tall trees to the narrow street. He moved little and pain painted his face.

It was here in the family home, in the fall of the year, that Joyce was engaged in caring for her dying father, a man full of kindness and joy of living, now waiting for the end of his time. All we could do was wait and make him comfortable, as the cancer ate him away.

After he went to a hospice facility near us in Arlington, I was able to see him more often as he withered away. One morning Joyce visited him and discovered he was tied down to the bed, against the family's wishes. It was an imprisonment that reinforced the duality of life and death. It was a terrible thing to see, yet there was something ennobling about a man struggling through sedation for life so actively he had to be shackled.

* * *

All that is familiar and brought me happiness is wasting away. I am starved of memory and not even the calendar can inform me of the day or week, while the year 2000 comes to a close.

The house on Ivy Street filled Joyce with energy and eagerness and she reached out to recover dreams laid aside in Delaware. Before we met, she had studied art at the Corcoran in Washington, D.C., and she decided to continue her studies at a local collage that also had classes in history, another subject of interest. To do this she gave up her part-time job and I went to work at an art supply store not far from Ivy Street where I had worked earlier making picture frames.

Before long an old Arlington school turned into a center for artists to work. When there was an opening, Joyce settled in, riding her old bicycle the few blocks to her studio. It was a wonderful, quiet place, full of interesting people and ideas. Unfortunately it was not the best place to sell art.

After a few years, a large building on the Alexandria waterfront, a former U.S. government document storage center, opened with the purpose of showing art and artists. It was called the Torpedo Factory Art Center and there was room for more than 150 artists. Several of the artists from the Arlington Art Center took studios there, and Joyce soon followed.

Joyce likes cats in twos, and soon after Una's arrival an artist with a studio down the hall from Joyce's in the Torpedo Factory Art Center told her of the litter of kittens his cat had delivered. One day he brought them to work in a box for Joyce to see. She came home with a tiny ball of almost white fur with a dark head. She was called Sabina. As she aged, the dark head was unchanged, but the lovely white coat turned dusty and her tail became black; only her belly retained its kitty white.

The new cats were so small we worried we might step on them, but they turned out to be nimble and flexible. The cats grew quickly, and before long they were climbing ladders. They had no apparent sense of fear but their antics often brought parental reproaches. As they grew older, we noticed differences in the cats, and they became individuals with personalities and obviously held on to memories of us and the rest of their world.

When you can't remember yesterday, memory is your only link to who you are. What happens when memory is gone? Alzheimer's finishes you off.

❁

PETULANT WHITE AND red lights hurry along the night dark roads leading away from the new twenty-story tombstones along the streets where I walk. Morning and night I walk over sidewalks, trying to remember what occupied the land when I was young. The Redskins football practice field is now a bus barn.

Car dealers are disappearing and where they were, tall buildings for business and apartments fill the space with lengthening shadows. Across the street a huge hole in the earth sits calmly while it is filled by early-morning men. Cold and wet they stoop and spit, erecting yet another office building to shadow places that once gave meaning to my life.

Places around me are dying as surly as am I, making way for a new world in which to fornicate, defecate and tell stories that buoy and sink our lives.

My exchange with the world brings life into the dead places in me.

*   *   *

My life slows as living becomes more arduous and memory loss becomes more severe. It never occurred to me how memory was so important to the smooth working of daily life.

What are the ingredients of a breakfast I have made for years? Writing small familiar words becomes a time-consuming struggle.

I can see and feel the familiar but it is presented in what appears new without any possibility to scan memory and plumb the past for all it once contained.

I can feel the hair on my head. Without a mirror, it feels like a memory to touch.

Fleeting memories of the past curl around my empty-ing brain, searching for a past to remember; any little scrap will do.

❋

ALL PLEASURE HAS DISAPPEARED, even the idea of enjoyment is gone. In its place there is numbness. I wake in the night and find I have an erection but there is no pleasure in watching it move and harden. There is no joy in my life, only difficulty slings at me. Almost any memory disappears as fast as it comes to life. I live in a world of surprises and fogs of fear.

The interiors and exteriors of the world flash before me but I cannot find ways to open them. I remain outside looking in, unable to open the past. My brain creaks through a world becoming unknown to itself.

Simple things are difficult and every minute is a frustrating struggle. I worry I will drive off and forget where I am going and why I am in the car. I want to crawl out of my body and dis-appear into a world I can understand, move to a country where language does not sizzle before my eyes and flicker in the midnight dark. Sometimes I think I have the mind of a baby and I slip into a world of unfamiliar streets. At other times, I float in a place of opulent emptiness.

As my world fades, Joyce's seems to change, too. She swims in hours of television and slaps herself over not completing things. She too is falling apart, not from disease but from sorrow and frustration, watching the man she loves disappear before her eyes.

> In the winter of my years, I see the dark birds circling the brick office building outside my window. They float and dive as a unit. This large flock appears to be searching for something lost, as am I.

❧

STILL OUT OF steady work during the second spring we lived in the house on Ivy Street, I began to take seriously an idea rolling around in my head. Where it came from, I know not, but it could have come from those long-ago summer vacation trips to Iowa.

I eagerly sniffed the edges of the world of farming, but not horticulture as it was normally practiced. This farming did not use tractors and require many acres of land. My dream was to grow potted plants in the minimal space in my backyard.

One of the first things I did was go to the county courthouse to see if my backyard dreams had legal backing. While Arlington had lost the agricultural look it had in the early nineteen hundreds, it retained a number of laws permitting individuals to grow and sell crops from their property, no matter how large the space.

I started out with common plants. It was soon evident that competition was heavy at that level. I looked deeper into the garden and found herbs, about which little had been written at the time, and what was published was full of inaccuracy and witchcraft.

Herbs were easily grown from small cuttings or seeds, and they didn't require acreage. I thought many of these varieties, unknown to American gardeners, would easily sell to gardeners anxious for a wider variety of unusual, edible plants. Eventually I became a specialist, searching for new varieties and creating a few of my own.

Although my father was dead, I remembered how he worked with his hands remodeling and working in the yard. Memories of watching him work with his hands after work made it easy for me to build the confidence I needed to start the project.

I had no idea how long it would take, or how many detours would be required before I reached my goal of farming my backyard for a living. I watched my father plant gardens in the spring, along with the other men in the neighborhood when I was a child, and, if anything, growing a garden is child's play, just a few years away from making mud pies.

Going into business was more serious than a simple garden. It required knowledge and skill not yet acquired. My days in the Library of Congress reading room filled many gaps in my education, but every plot of a farm, even a small one, has variations in soil texture and type. This is why many growers use greenhouses, convenient sunny work spaces where the environment is manipulated. No matter how much I studied or how expert I became there remained secrets only years of hard work and curiosity could unearth.

Starting small was smart, but tiny was all I had. I spent almost nothing on the first cold frames I built to protect the young plants from early cold, spring weather. Joyce's father brought scrap pieces of wood from one of his building jobs. He also brought bales of straw. His largest contribution was the group of old windows he salvaged from a home remodeling job.

With his scrap wood, I built open-topped boxes about two feet high on the side that faced the sun and, behind it, sides three feet high, giving the cold frame a slope to allow water to run off the short structures and also to allow for the opening of the old windows that were attached to the high back of the low structure. Easy opening of the top of the cold frame made it simple to regulate heat on warm days in spring and summer.

To sell plants, I constructed a lean-to between the house and the west side of the property line. The other side of the house was not useful for selling but it came in handy for holding plants ready to sell.

Early in the spring, after several gloriously warm days, I inspected the cold frames and found tiny black snakes sunning themselves on the decomposing straw bales. I was surprised. I had not seen snakes at any time around the house. As little black snakes wiggled out of spring's warmth I realized the bales of straw sitting on a construction site before being moved to my backyard came loaded with unwanteds. It was unfortunate I had no taste for young snake flesh.

That first year I put signs on the busy street a few steps from our house promoting my little backyard business. The first customers wanted to bargain over the 25-cent plants in paper cups. We held firm, and by the end of the day, all our plants were sold.

A few days later I got a job in an art store where I had worked earlier and we began to have a more solvent way of life.

> Sometimes memory thinks faster than I do. At other times it is slow and turbulent. Yet again, remembering things is almost impossible. What day is it? What month? What happened yesterday?

I walked along the sidewalk next to a deep hole, dug to begin yet another high-rise building designed to generate money for someone and destroy a place of modest beauty. A young woman and her mother with a small child in a stroller stopped me. I thought they were lost and needed directions.

We are headed for the shelter tonight, she said, but we don't have money for food. She was nervous and embarrassed.

The wind was icy but not as frosty as it would be in a few hours. I gave the young woman $25 and wished I had more to give the three of them. The county shelter is a crowded place of last resort, yet there are many homeless people who eschew its winter warmth and bundle up against warm buildings instead.

On my three-mile walk I pass four churches standing on large expansive manicured lawns. Six days a week the churches are empty and locked or filled with basements of day care children. One day a week they open their doors for a few hours to talk of holiness and the importance of living a Christian life.

My birthday is January 5, today. Before long I will be a scuffling, old child, a year before toppling into the sixties, if I am lucky.

The cold frames were a good way to start a shoestring business but they were not useful year-round. Before long I began to think of greenhouses, structures with stand-up space and heaters. I liked the idea of a place where I didn't have to work in bad weather throughout the entire year.

An advertisement in one of the many grower magazines I received caught my eye. It offered a glass greenhouse of modest size with vented roofs and sliding front doors. It was moderately priced and easily expanded in length by bolting a new section onto the existing one. To begin, I ordered two new sections.

The day the delivery truck arrived I was at work and the driver dumped everything on the front lawn. The glass was carefully packed and in wood boxes. They were so heavy, I had to unpack them where they stood. I marveled at how the driver was able to unload them by hand. It took several hours to move all the glass and other equipment. I was panting and sore but I was eager to get to work.

The greenhouse was constructed by bolting two sections together. The structure went in a straight line toward the neighbor's garage, an attempt to give her an open view without having to see greenhouses. The design of the new greenhouses called for the metal pieces to sit on two-by-eights. The entire forty-foot length was dug creating a level bed for the two by eights. Getting everything plumb was important. Francesco helped me all he could but he had homework and two newspaper routes at the time. I loved the sliding door until winter arrived and I learned about the power water created when it turned to ice on the inside and outside of the metal uprights.

Once the greenhouse was up I installed a large electric heater and two long benches to hold potted plants.

> Memories float to the top of consciousness, swirling and diving. I try to catch them but they slip away and I am left empty and in tears.

The greenhouse has been kind to me in a bitter way. It was the necessity that kept me alive and the family together, but it was costly. It was like putting my dreams of writing in a safe deposit box so I could stay alive. It was a choice I made freely under helpless coercion.

※

MY LIFE, once orderly and tranquil, is unraveling.

I have forgotten how to set the thermostat to govern the heat of the house in winter.

We have already installed signs on the outside of kitchen cabinets to inform me what I will find in them. The big problem is I sometimes don't understand the sign for some time.

It takes longer almost every day to remember the makeup of

my breakfast. Before long everything will have to be labeled for me as I lose my mind.

I become agitated easily from frustration over little things. It was easily handled a few years ago, but now a bomb swells inside me until I explode.

I have difficulty remembering the names of friends.

How long will it be before I am imprisoned here, trembling, forgetful and without the memory of who I am or who I used to be?

As memory slips away, I resort to scribbling memory on folded slips of paper. My memory is carried on quarter notes, folded on slips of paper stuffed in my shirt pockets.

I turned around and saw my cat Sabina behind me. She was watching the letters pile up on the computer screen as I write this. She does not know what they are but she knows something is there moving before her eyes. She asks no more of me than to make the letters jump and career forward and backward. Movement is enough, as it often is for us as we watch a movie, a car race, or a basketball or football game. Motion is a way of knowing you are alive.

The long, tapered, silver bucket filled with passengers glides out of the clouds as it heads for National Airport. Birds romp on top of the firehouse across the street, gliding and flapping their wings on this shivering morning.

Can I stay in touch with my memories while I sleep?

Hoarfrost clings to the brown grass. Tree limbs are bare, with stately, thin branches. In the morning, light strikes the bare limbs and the air trembles. The days of change and death approach.

*   *   *

A sky of pleated clouds is scudding by. The sparkle once in my eyes is dull and vacant. I stare into eternity and see nothing.

There are many moments when my eyes see but there is a numbness in my brain that is not connected to what I see. I see but I remain numbed, staring without thinking.

Approximately four million Americans have Alzheimer's disease but the illness touches many more. In a 1993 survey, 19 million Americans said they had a family member with the disease and 37 million said they knew someone with the disease. More than 7 of 10 people with Alzheimer's live at home and nearly 75 percent of their care is provided by families and friends.

—The Alzheimer's Association

These cold winter mornings send my cat Una into the bathroom where she huddles for warmth close to the old, pealing radiator. It is there I find her when I join her in the warmth of a new day. Una quietly sneaks out of the bathroom as I shave. She knows the shower comes next and she cannot abide the sound and smell of water.

Whispers of humanity hide along the ether.

My life is dissolving into an unhappy scream as I slide into a time of anger at little, helpless things I can no longer control.

I wade in too deep and come up spluttering.

I am almost useless except to make others angry with me while the hopes of a lifetime disintegrate into unhappiness and whispers.

Heavy clouds move in and leave me stumbling and lost in the thick fog of my mind.

I am coming to a place in my faltering life where the unknown is yesterday and today is filled with repressed memory.

I am becoming a lousy piece of meat for the ones I love the most.

I am helpless in the face of death that comes from behind me with the flash and whisper of a knife.

It is not the sepulcher where the hurt lives wagging its finger at me, it is the twisting mental messages that cause the worst bewilderment.

Some days I know only my cat is aware of what I am going through, and she welcomes a tender pat of her soft purr. The slow movement of my hand through the cat's soft fur is enough to get me through the day sane, if there is such a thing any more.

In the end, the tactile, loving touch says all that need be said.

Sparkling lights blink through the night sky, airliners compete with slow planets and winking asteroids.

Shadows of another life flicker in the corners of my eyes. There are fantasies yet to be visited, mysteries in dark nights without dreams.

Before slumber takes over, my head on the pillow is filled with standing people, one in each blink of my polarized eyelids. They stand stiff in the old-fashioned way, these visions, standing for a photograph. The individuals in these simple poses wear plain or fancy garments. These are images from a stereopticon like my Grandma Davis showed me one day in the little sewing room off the big, bright kitchen in her house in Eldora, Iowa.

Even in the long-ago era of the stereopticon, images were used to capture time as it slipped away. We capture our age and our lives with different equipment today, but the urge to hold a living moment forever remains strong.

Now I want to lash out in a vain attempt to stop the movement of time so I can hold my days forever and drift in a melancholy pool. I wait anxiously for a little more time.

*   *   *

In the quiet street gutter, emptied of leaves by a brisk overnight wind, tiny, tan stones still rattle in the wind as the impotent sun smiles on the world.

I found myself becoming silent last night as we ate a late supper with Francesco and Tammy. After I checked the kitchen where Tammy was putting the finishing touches on the meal, I turned off the world and went into what pretends to be my memory. Mentally I faded away while the world rolled on, as water carries me away into places of which I have never spoken.

When I became conscious of the world again, I was sitting in Francesco's living room watching the flames in the beautiful stone fireplace. I was barefoot as my son requires of those who enter his house, and Joyce was sitting next to me. In the background the television winked, tripping over itself on the way to oblivion sometime after midnight. I did not mean this behavior to be a subtle insult, if anyone actually noticed it.

I cannot explain my silence or understand why I sometimes prefer its empty appetite to the rustle of the world. These are new things inhabiting my secret places. I know they come though doors of death but I do not understand their language nor the reason for their presence. My silence did not come from fear of becoming tangled in vocabulary. For many long moments, I was as empty as the chilly wind outside.

As the fireplace crackled I disappeared from time to time, although I remained visible. Enjoying this new freedom of walking around with an unhinged brain while sitting in a soft chair put me at a distance from other people. Silence shrouds my mind these frosty, sad, cold days of autumn. Icy sparkling nights carry me to new places where street gutters are full of tiny, tan stones rattling in a low wind of impotent smiles.

*   *   *

The cold numbs my fingers as I sit on the curbstone,
scribbling my life away. Where once my dreams swelled,
there is now emptiness and frozen tears.

In the early days after I was diagnosed with Alzheimer's, the
worst was forgetting. There was allowance for humor, such as
the night when I prepared dinner twice. Now as the third year
with the disease draws near, there is less levity in me and the
way I look at the world, although laughter is not entirely gone.

Unhappiness shows itself often, especially when there is a
group in the house. Amid chatter, I am silent. I sit with my
elbows on my knees and stare straight ahead. My mind is nearly
empty in these moments; I could be asleep except my eyes are
open. Gone are the days when my brain was bright and full of
clever offerings that bubbled against one another.

I can hear the dull talk around me, but I am not there in the
room mentally; I float in a world emptied of sentience. Nothing
exists for short moments except the air around me. I could as
well be a statue.

Alzheimer's has become an angry spot that never stops rub-
bing me bare. The disease is a spit in the face, a knuckle jab to
the groin, a prison sentence from nowhere. I seethe with private
anger I dare not expose except in private moments alone.

I had dreams last night in which fire destroyed my
mind, leaving me cleansed and alone. When I awoke a
cold sun was shining and a brisk wind slashed at my coat.
I can still laugh at the cold and shake hands with the sun.

This morning I discovered I could see different still scenes
before my shut eyes. I moved from slide to slide by blinking my
eyes. This was different from earlier manifestations of seeing
things with my eyes closed.

The hallucination took place in my bedroom. The blinds were closed and little light filtered into the room. I lay on my bed and shut my eyes. I saw a still life of an old stereopticon like my grandmother's. I shut my eyes harder, hoping to eliminate images and go to black; instead another blurred image appeared in still life. I did not recognize the images on the screens before my eyes.

With my memory slowly crumbling, I thought these new apparitions might be an attempt by my brain to bring me a disheveled past in a novel way. I have no idea why the images hovered in a mist, making it impossible for me to recognize the place and the people shown. This is the way Alzheimer's plays with me.

My mind is a-twitter with echoes of spent words that persist in bobbing to the surface of my consciousness and licking the edge of memory. Yet in a few seconds it is flashed away, leaving bewildered emptiness.

A dry leaf throbs on the sidewalk this gray November day.

An angry, disheveled man shouts at cars as he crosses the street. A chill, not from the cold, runs through me. I look over my shoulder several times and he continuous to berate some unseen antagonist. He blows up again and crosses the street flaying with shouted words a make-believe antagonist. Finally I am far enough away and his explosive temper is out of sight and sound. I realize I have a pocket of anger like his and I could be him some fine explosive day.

A civilization should be more than the sum of money and pleasure.

I don't know what I will write, if anything, until I head out for my three-mile walk. The turnabout is usually in the damp early mornings, along a winding concrete sidewalk paralleling a busy thoroughfare.

When I near the walk's finish, ideas often flood my mind, leaving me on the street side scribbling before the words and ideas vanish and are lost forever. Usually I capture enough words to embellish and expand the few sentences that started the whole affair. Life in the streets with cars slipping a few feet away fires my creative juices. The words caught on the walk usually provide hours of fun during the day as I move them around and escort them to the paragraphs marching down the cluttered piece of white paper.

In the last few days, a huge crane was installed half a mile away. It is a giant piece of equipment, strong in ways I can understand. It stands upright and lifts weight no man can. This skinny piece of construction equipment is now the tallest thing within sight. Behind it, and miles away, airplanes flutter down onto the runways at Washington National Airport. With all the tall buildings and those coming, even the sky is crowded outside my window.

Building these tall office buildings and sky-high apartments has been going on for many years. The county fathers decided we needed a "downtown," a sharp modern look to shake its old image as a pleasant, happy place to live. Now it has the charm of a dog fight, and it is not yet over.

A few blocks from our house on Ivy Street, an entire road is roped off for destruction, the new slow process of urban evolution. Close up, my part of Arlington is a city of huge sticks in deep yellow earth, announced by signs that say, "Build to suit, office/retail". When we moved here thirty years ago everything but the schools were the height of a two-story house or less.

The latest site near us was a parking lot near a Metro station. Now it is another yellow hole, a cemetery for underground life.

Buildings are coming at us from right and left and the soul of the place is changing rapidly before my eyes. Rank visual emptiness bounces against the pleasant souls of the past, now buried in a cemetery of sorrow.

I remember Arlington as a small village with low houses and small lots with thick stands of trees. These memories, butting up against the new reality of change, have set me daydreaming of moving to the country where the earth still looks the way it did fifty years ago in the part of Arlington with no sidewalks where I grew up.

As I walked back from looking at the crane close up, I passed an architect's office on the ground floor of a building. I looked in the window and saw a man in a blue shirt talking to a younger man sitting at a desk. The man standing with the blue shirt has flipped his red tie over his shoulder.

> As I pass the bank, the clock ticks with the sound of a
> club hitting dirt, agitating the weight of time as it marks
> its rhythmic measure of death one minute after the other.
> The sound of the clock brought back the chatter of chil-
> dren and my childhood, but their memories were still
> and liquid, a state impossible to interpret.

Christmas Day, 2000. I am working today, tapping at this keyboard with little time left, in an attempt to understand who I was and what is left. I have little chance at knocking this computer many more days. I am up against the wall with little time before I hang up my passport and shiver into the last time of my life.

My life creaks toward childhood. I have lost my ability to do simple math; adding and subtracting has befuddled me for months. Although I am able to type, about every other word is misspelled and I fight a losing battle to retain vocabulary. Words tell us who we are and where we've been. Words make us sad and happy. To lose word-making skills is to compromise a large part of what makes us who we are. Words provide details of the world in which we live and a way to understand what goes on. At some point, not far off, I will not be able to kiss Joyce or enjoy Francesco's jokes.

All day I wrestled with the feeling of being empty, a man drained of humanity and meaning who stares into the void in helpless anger without courting comprehension. I have slowly become a useless vessel in the hands of Alzheimer's.

Joyce and I have talked several times about taking trips, flying away to happy, interesting foreign lands and unusual places. I see a man with Alzheimer's swirl off to play and travel, a last chance to carry on and have fun. It is something I have never done and the idea has an almost irresistible charm. Yet, I hem and haw and roll my head in the sand. We go nowhere.

What I have been unable to tell Joyce clearly is that I don't want to wander outside my deteriorating brain. With the onset of Alzheimer's, I saw new revelations and visited places I had never been. They have turned out to be as useful, frightening, pleasant and beautiful as anything I could have wished. The real reason we haven't gone anywhere is that I am afraid of getting lost. I need the familiar around me to give me comfort and stability. I am at such a tender point in life now that I worry when I head out for the grocery store five blocks away. I get angry if a chair is moved in the house.

I wanted to chart this world of memory I've discovered inside my brain but I am beginning the exploration too late. The fires of Alzheimer's have nearly destroyed my short-term memory. My long-term memory is left battered; trying to find moments of the past is like fishing with a dull, rusting hook without bait.

New Year's Eve. Sabina rolls on the floor in her gray, pleated fir. Afterward she rests her back feet at an angle to allow her to take off in a cat's instant. Her favorite place to sit is in front of the kitchen refrigerator, where heat blows gently from under the machine while she stretches out to enjoy it in a contemplative peace.

After stoking up heat, her next favorite occupation is coaxing me to play with her. For this she requires a specific string, either black or white, about three feet long. My joy is to work the string under her nose where she can pounce and chew it ragged. When she tires of this, she instructs me to swish the string back and forth so she can chase it. Thus does her day slip by from chair in the dining room to lunch. After lunch a snooze in my workroom upstairs, where she sleeps in a blue chair over which colorful old towels have been placed to keep the chair clean. She wakes when the outdoors darkens silently. Soon she is on her way to the kitchen and begins screaming for food.

Sabina is a gentle cat, made deaf by a careless veterinarian. In time she has overcome her handicap with powerful understanding of her place in the world. She is talkative but not understandable by our ears. She sticks to a routine as finely honed as mine, demanding food at exacting moments during the day. We understand each other, all that is necessary for anybody to get along in the world.

❧

I WAS DESPERATE for money. The plant business was still small and seasonal. I asked Francesco's *Washington Star* delivery man about getting a job on a truck like his. He said there were often jobs available, especially for substitute drivers. I applied and soon had a $200-a-week job, more than I had ever been paid.

The first week was fun. There was a procession of three

experienced delivery men to show me the ropes. I was the substitute for each of them. I learned how each man conducted his deliveries, where the delivery van was kept, and what I was expected to do. It turned out to be a lot more than dropping bundled newspapers at carriers' homes.

My first surprise was delivering newspapers to stores, as well as to the kids who delivered the papers after school. On one route there was even a special delivery to Dulles Airport, well over an hour from where I lived and in unfamiliar territory.

Most of the drivers did not take their delivery trucks home. They drove to the area where they worked and picked up their truck where it was left the previous day. Most delivery vans were tucked out of the way in shopping centers or friendly gasoline stations.

As a substitute driver I learned three different routes. Two of them were close to an hour away. The third was in a rough area with many boarded-up houses covering parts of Arlington and Alexandria. It was in an area I frequented when I was trying to make my way as a potter after Joyce and I were married.

The word "carriers" was always used to identify the children who delivered the newspapers to homes. It was a way to blur the reality of child exploitation. Part of my job after dropping bundles of papers was to circle around, make sure the kids delivered their papers, and once a month collect the money the kids received from their customers.

When I knocked on a carrier's door to pick up the money he had collected for the *Star*, there were often angry parents to greet me. When the bill came, it was often greater than their child was able to collect from his customers and the newspaper insisted on prompt payment. The children were expected to collect what was owed the *Star*, less a small amount for themselves. Many of the carriers' parents expressed unhappiness, calling the *Star* cheats and extortioners.

I had a collision with theft eventually. A few times I collected money for the regular drivers. Instead of taking the money bag with me to the house as I was told to do, I left it in the truck without locking the doors. I would only be a moment. When I returned, the money, a substantial sum, was gone. The company rules were that I had to make good on the money. It was much more than a single payday and I reported the theft with trepidation. The kids on the street knew who stole the money but were afraid to tell. The regular driver, more familiar with the kids and the area, found the culprit and retrieved the money from a manhole.

Monday through Friday the *Star* was an afternoon newspaper. On Saturday and Sunday it turned into a morning newspaper. Friday, Saturday and Sunday were the toughest days. Friday was difficult because it was important to get home early and it was almost impossible to get home before eight P.M. All the drivers were out delivering missed papers and collecting money until late most week nights.

Saturday the newspaper was delivered in the morning and that meant I had to get up around one A.M., leaving me about three to four hours' sleep before it was time to get ready to get out to the delivery truck and drop papers to the carriers by five A.M. Sunday was not as bad as long as I went to bed early enough to get up at one A.M. again. Sometimes it appeared there was no life outside the *Washington Star.*

Often I got to see Francesco, and Joyce, still watching television when I got up a little after midnight to prepare for Saturday's and Sunday's newspaper drops. When I finished the Saturday drops, I drove back to the house and picked up Francesco, who had been out delivering papers. We headed for breakfast with another driver before delivering papers that carriers had skipped. Francesco was fond of these meetings, but my head was swimming from lack of sleep. When I eventually quit the job, I think we both missed those moments together in the early morning eating breakfast and delivering newspapers.

Before long I learned that my new job on a delivery truck was hard and dangerous, something I never saw as a kid carrier in an earlier time. The job involved a lot more than kicking bundles of newspapers out of an open truck. A number of times I got lost and ended up wandering around unfamiliar territory, but my memory was good enough to help me find my way back.

One Sunday morning darkness and thick fog hugged me. The fog was so thick I got out of the truck to see where I was several times. It was frightening but as daylight came it was easier to see. This occurred during a time all of Northern Virginia was under a rolling blackout. Some areas had no electricity at night, others none during the day. In Reston no convenience stores had electricity. Fortunately, my greenhouse business was on the same blackout schedule and during cold nights the greenhouses were warmed by electric heaters.

The worst thing that happened was trying to put on snow chains when I got stuck on an icy cul-de-sac outside Reston. I pulled a muscle putting on the chains. The pain lingered and I went to the company's doctor, who sent me to a place that warmed my back and gave me pain pills. In time I recovered, but I realized this was not the kind of job I wanted, and I went back to struggling with herb plants and greenhouses.

Mysterious deep red contrails hang from the sky, long and flirtatious, weeping against the setting sun.

Journalism kept a bear hug on me and I jumped at the chance to return when I heard the weekly *Arlington News* was looking for an editor. I walked the two blocks from home to the newspaper's office. I had a fistful of clippings and asked for the job. I was lucky, or so I thought. I was asked to start the next day as managing editor.

The newspaper's office was not as crowded as some where I had worked, but it had a hurried look. On my first day of work,

I learned that the last editor had walked out because he wasn't paid. The paper was so impecunious nobody was paid except essential people. I was promised pay and I actually received a check once.

Money was not my motivation. I wanted to write and change the world, something my fledgling plant business did not offer. Newspapers were my dream from the time I was fourteen. I thought I could have a fling on this little paper between Christmas and the end of March when I planned to open to sell plants at the nursery on Ivy Street.

The second payday I received only part of what was due. By then it made no difference; I was digging dirt right and left and delivering the paper. Then one Monday morning I walked to the newsroom and found it empty. Everything was gone and there was a large hole in the floor where the equipment had been wrenched down two stories to a moving van. As the editor of the newspaper, I had scooped myself. I went home and started making calls to locate the new address.

Before long I discovered the newspaper office had moved to a warehouse near the railroad switching yard. I drove over to see whether I was the victim of a silent firing or whether they got out in such a hurry they didn't remember the new editor.

The new home of the *Arlington News* was a damp, cold warehouse. I found the publisher's office, such as it was, at the end of a long, dark, damp corridor. I was shown to a lovely little office with a door, much nicer than the previous location. From what I could ascertain, the landlord of the previous office was unhappy without rent payments.

There was no heat in the new location, not a good situation for January in Northern Virginia. Mary was running the paper and she located small heaters for her office and mine. Smudge pots, or a close relative, were used to heat the rest of the warehouse.

Wandering around the newspaper building one afternoon I

discovered a large open area in the warehouse where hundreds of bundles of newspapers lay undelivered. In several cases it appeared the entire press run was dumped. I reflected for a couple of days and then told Mary I wasn't coming back.

Soon after I left, the newspaper permanently folded. There was still time to send catalogs to my spring plant customers, and I went back to the greenhouse for good. I understood the land and the seeds, and the sun and the rain. I knew how they worked together and I felt at home in this small place in my backyard.

Every morning I awake in an unfamiliar thicket of blankets with a faint recollection there was a past but I have only the faintest idea of yesterday.

❋

The gutter is full of dun-colored leaves, detritus of summer's life. An icy wind enters the street and the chattering leaves rise and dance into the air. Memories of the past, vague shadows now with little stamina, race along with the leaves, weaving a tapestry at once warm and nippy. The wind-like memories whistle through my fingers, unseen but felt, even as they hide from the reaper. I grab at the twisting memories but I am no longer quick enough to capture these forgotten moments of joy and wonder.

We are all homeless animals, wandering in search of something.

I am on the edge of turning over all bill-paying chores to Joyce. With a good list I can still do the grocery shopping but the frustration ratio has become rather higher than it has ever been. Yesterday was the worst.

I lost my ability to add and subtract without a machine some time ago. Trying to do it in my head as I used to is now a screaming match within myself. This fight with a failing brain brings tears to my eyes and exhausts me physically. Alzheimer's eats me away in little increments, stealing here, bombing there, until there is little left to enjoy in life.

There are places carrying strong memories, and in their presence the past returns with vividness and tears. I entered such a place yesterday, a little park with a tennis court on which I once played badly.

All around this park were pieces of me. I walked along the helpless little stream, fishless and no longer polluted, as it zigzagged through the trees bordering it. I wept at the sound of water running over mossy stones.

The water was clear and it reflected the leafy trees and the blue sky. I looked at the sparkling water and saw a place important to my adolescence. It was here in a time with a halting path that the course of my life was settled. From the secrets of this park, poetry came to me and left its mark, and I made promises unkept.

Where there is now a towpath full of mothers pushing baby strollers, a railroad once slowly rumbled into my life. Here again in my imagination were the large, dark, heavy trains moving slowly with ever-dwindling rolling stock. Now even the little house along the tracks where a switchman stayed is gone, erased from time but not memory.

In was in this park I played joyously, often by myself, before the bolder dust was green. It was a time when the little falls welcomed the water but it bubbled with pollution and the bottom was filled with stones but they were often blurred by the sewage the little creek carried.

I looked up the steep hill and saw the backyard that nurtured me and I remembered the swamp where little peepers serenaded spring, while the freight trains passed slowly. I yearn to walk up the steep hill and wander through the backyard full of memories lost so long ago. Would the present occupants understand if I told them I wanted one last look at a link of my life before I died of Alzheimer's?

I walked along the length of the little park and more memories displayed themselves. It was in this place I grew into manhood and threw away the humble places dearest to me. The trees are taller now and the still neighborhood of my adolescence looks the same. The memories of those who lived there in my childhood now haunt the place that was once mine.

Maybe the earth remembered me as I walked alone along little Four Mile Run as the daffodils stretched and brought forth heads of yellow, brighter than the rough soils from which they came.

THERE WAS A bell in the kitchen to alert me to temperature problems in my backyard greenhouses. One icy night a little before midnight the bell started to clatter, sending fear through my body. It was very cold and there was little I could do to provide alternative heat. I had only one emergency gas heater, which required electricity.

The temperatures in each of the four greenhouses was close to freezing and there was no ready explanation for it. In a panic, I called the gas company. In a few hours, a crew was at the house. The cause of the cold greenhouses was lack of enough gas flowing though the pipes. When the lines were put underground I had not realized I needed to contact the gas company to change the amount of gas flowing through the pipes.

A long line of geese congregate in a dark line against a dusty, pebbled sky, honking out of sight over leafless trees. The bareness of winter freezes tears in my eyes.

I keep things long after their useful lives expire. It is a way I hold on to the past and compare it with the present.

Now the little room where I work overflows with unusable objects, clutter of my past, tottering above the abyss, as I laugh and cry my way through days sparkling with forgetfulness.

I am on the edge of tears. There is nowhere to hide, as I did when a child. In those early days I wrapped myself in a private world where I was in control, captain of a spaceship circling a new galaxy. Now wind rattles dry leaves and I slip into my childhood secret world, but there are no galaxies left to explore, only uncontrollable tears coursing down my cheeks.

Snow has thickened the cold air this Saturday and turned the world into a soupy mist. So thick is it that the huge crane, usually visible from my office window, is a bare shadow of itself. Even a freshet of snow like this has been a long time coming and I am anxious to walk through it, enshrouding my presence and hiding the tears covering my face.

I do a lot of walking but it is always along familiar sidewalks. My route takes me three miles, back and forth to my house in a circle. The fevered moment of fear that greets the bewildered is yet to make itself known, but I feel it is near.

I have moments when my mind is lost momentarily and I am left with a feeling of hurt, fear and bewilderment, so powerful my breath becomes broken and there is fear in my pocket. I am thankful I do not yet live in the strange world without signs; familiar places and friendly faces still exist in my world.

To prepare for the moment when the world becomes strange and I begin wandering without meaning or knowledge, Joyce bought silver bracelets for each of us from the Alzheimer's Association. The top of my sparkling bracelet carries the organization's Safe Return logo. On the other side of the bracelet are words that chilled me when I read them:

MEMORY IMPAIRED
TO HELP TOM
CALL 1-800-572-1122
(The next line carries my ID number.)

Reading these words brought tears to my eyes, and still does many days later as I write this. This is yet another reminder of my Alzheimer's-ravaged brain. On a normal day, I have hundreds of such encounters. Having a bracelet on my wrist is further confirmation of my plight. I hope this bracelet remains a piece of jewelry and is not needed to identify me on some lonely street corner.

I have never been a man fond of jewelry. The bracelet provided by the association is handsome and unintrusive, and I have grown to like it. The information on the bracelet helps a police officer identify me quickly and report my whereabouts and where I live. It is of a much better quality than the Sky King ring I got in a cereal box as a child.

Secrets unmasked: Why is there a bird in our refrigerator? Joyce found the bird dead some years ago and froze it to make it useful as a model for paintings.

Pigeons roost on a large apartment building, warming themselves in the parsimonious warmth of an overcast winter day. There are other buildings all around but no other structure has birds sunning themselves.

The birds march around on the sharp incline of the roof with haughty precision. They politely giggle for position on the roof, sliding sideways and then moving back and forth. The nervous pigeons cluster in the place where a shaft of sunlight hits and warms the roof.

Across the street an Arlington police officer sits in his clearly marked car. He is waiting for speeders. I walk about a block before I hear the siren. A man in a beat-up, colorful car meets a side-street cop.

※

ONE NIGHT IN early fall, after the cool night air turned black, Joyce and I heard a loud and angry conversation outside. Through the window we saw in the dim streetlights two people arguing at the used-car lot on the other side of 10th Street.

The shouting continued and I looked out the window again. All I saw was the little narrow road in front of the house and the tall streetlight next to the lot.

Things calmed down before there was a knock at the door. I opened the door to a young woman with tears coursing down her cheeks. She was breathless and obviously frightened.

Are you all right, I asked.

It's my boyfriend, she said. He wants to kill me.

Come in quickly, I said.

She came in and stood in the vestibule. I locked the front door. Joyce came into the room to see what was going on. The woman told her through tears what she told me.

I'll call the police, I said.

No, please don't, she said.

When I pressed her for a reason for not making the call, she stepped toward the door.

If you go, use the back door, I said.

The light at the back door illuminated her back as she walked down the steps. Greenhouses covered the backyard and she slipped into the darkness between the high fence and a tall greenhouse.

For another hour, we heard scattered shouting in the trembling dark.

I see a white-haired man with a protruding belly a block ahead of me. He stares into a huge hole, nearly a block square, as a new building takes shape. He appears to be watching the men, made small by the great depth of the hole, scurrying around in the icy air deep in the ground below. Work becomes a spectator sport at a certain age.

※

MY LIFE IS guided by introspection. I took care of myself and tried to eat right. I thought these things were worthy and would obtain for me a long life. I adopted this life after I watched my parents die young, painful deaths, my father of a bad heart, my mother of cancer. After they died and the tears dried, I tried to do things to mitigate my chances of dying the way they did. I looked at my father's parents and saw hard work and long lives. I tried to follow in their footsteps.

It was a bewildering surprise when the doctor, without much preamble, told me I had Alzheimer's, a word I never heard associated with anyone in my family. It helped to remember the hidden death my parents carried within them for so many years before it smashed them as they looked forward to a quiet retirement with grandchildren and travel.

Now I see that my parents unwittingly presented me with a surprise, an early death so novel it was hardly known when I was born, a disease only now being understood and not yet cured. The disease is called Alzheimer's, a death mark from faulty genes and often passed through generations. Until there is a cure, there is forever emptiness and haunted eyes.

A lonely blackbird balances on the electric line next to the porch. It rocks back and forth to steady itself. For a fleeting moment it is still. Suddenly it is airborne and out of sight, carried by the thing we cannot see, the air we breathe.

As I went to bed, seventeen koi whose bright colors left sparks in my eyes for years swam slowly in a little backyard pool. Before long snowflakes began to fall. By morning the earth was lightly covered with snow.

I was no longer the keen observer I was before Alzheimer's took up residence inside me. I wish I remembered what I learned many years ago about water, ice and soft snow, but I was no longer outfitted with a keen mind.

The next morning, I looked out the dining room window and saw both of our little ponds covered with thick white ice. My mind did not dig deep in my memory and bring up the danger for the fish.

I went to the basement to water a few flats of plants growing under lights. It was then that I saw the water.

It was snow, not rain, that came in the night. I ran upstairs and rushed out the back door. The first thing I saw was the frozen filter of the fish pool, holding a large number of koi, a fish known for its beautiful coloring.

The filter system was set up to draw water from one of the fish ponds. The water flows into the top of a long, fat, gray tube and is discharged at the bottom of the filter. The water rises through a series of different-sized stones to clean the water of contaminants. The cleaned water flows through a pipe back to the pool. But ice formed under the outlet and, instead of returning to the pond, it flowed over the side of the filter and eventually entered the basement. The little pond with the largest population of fish pumped out almost all its water, leaving the fish struggling to draw water over their gills and breathe.

I broke through the ice-covered pool and found fish swimming, but there were many lifeless bodies on the bottom of the pool. I pulled out dead koi, carefully putting them in a box. As soon as the dead fish were out, I began to refill the little pond and restarted the bubbler to increase the amount of air in the water. Taking dead koi you have raised out of a cold winter pond is nothing like picking a piece of fish at the market. It is a sad, bleary moment of sadness and anger.

A shroud hangs over my life and the lives of other beings killed by my forgetfulness. The earth is frozen hard, making it impossible to bury the dead bodies. It is not too late to shed tears. These deaths in the cold water of a late December remind me I should begin to think of myself as a handicapped person, owned by Alzheimer's, incapable of doing yesterday's things easily.

The air is thick with pleated snow, garlanded with memories of a small boy with his first sled, a Christmas present from Santa Claus.

Fifty-five years later the boy has grown into a man without the wish for snow. His memories, corrupted by Alzheimer's, are difficult to find with so many lost to the fire burning in his brain.

I FLEW TO Iowa to watch my grandmother die. She was the last of our Iowa tribe. I walked into the hospital and found her in a small space. When she saw me approach her bed, she began to chant, Tom, Tom, Tom. There was little else she could communicate this late in her life, at 103 years old. She was sick and dying, outliving her children and her husband and her home, a nest reached by a long stairway on which she went up and down the long steep incline with the help of a motorized contraption. Her house was filled with things from another era, plain old stuff she cherished for the memories it brought her.

Beside her now I saw a woman I no longer recognized, a short woman of whom I knew little, except from the stories she told from her childhood right up to the present. The only story that morning was the one she chanted, Tom, Tom, Tom, the chant of memory pushing tears into my eyes. It is a chant living inside me, a chant that haunts me as I walk slowly in her path.

I hoped her genes of longevity had been passed to me. I worried about the cancer of my dead sweet mother and the bad heart left to my lifeless father. Alzheimer's was a secret word in their day.

At night sometimes, I awake to hear my grandmother chanting for me, Tom, Tom, Tom. The voice is reedy and strained and I want to turn away and walk in a different place where there is life and a bright sun, but there is now noplace for me to go. I wait.

I see dark snow camped on brittle waves of leaves while a wicked wind whistles up my sleeves, sending shivers through my body. My body trembles. Is it from the cold or from uncontrollable emotion?

I HAVE BECOME emotional and find tears on my cheeks when I least expect them. Tears come without warning, choking speech. Things I cannot find quickly grow into uncontrollable explosions. The world is slipping from my grasp. Frustration is abundant and I am filled with anxiety.

Squeaky floorboards speak to me in the guttural language of Hades.

The powerful winter wind tickles me as it rattles storm windows.

My most recent deficit occurred a few days ago. As I was reading, I found it difficult to understand a word. I recognized the letters but they did not mean anything; my vocabulary shrinks every day. This is why I call Alzheimer's the slow incremental death. It is so quiet and subtle it goes almost unnoticed.

I awoke this morning full of panting anxiety, unable to remember whether I am supposed to meet Dan and Tom at the Loudoun farm or at the house in Arlington.

Yet, after all this, I can still remember why there is a pile of ice bags on the porch. The bags were put there for my birthday party January 5. It was such a party, packed with old friends and new, that I don't think I will ever forget it. At the least I want to be reminded of it. It was the best thing I can remember and I have Joyce to thank for it all, along with my friend Rick Tag and my sister, Mary Ann, and her large, useful family.

No matter good or bad, I am descending into another world, full of unknown streets which I will not be able to describe for you.

The sun arose this morning through a streaked sky etched with blood. Above empty streets the wind was brisk, and loneliness was as palpable as the screaming cold. I sit here wondering which way the words will blow.

As I turned the corner and started the last leg of my afternoon walk, I admired the emptiness of the streets. So empty were they I could easily leave the sidewalk and meander down the middle of the street, past the empty bus parked along the road waiting for ghost riders or for the time to leave and start another round-robin of boredom behind the wheel. These ghost streets are dry and kicked by debris with the smell of cold emptiness.

I was about three quarters of the way home when the chills began to weasel their way through the many layers of clothing I had wrapped around me to keep me warm. I looked to my right as I started to cross a street. Coming down the middle of a furtive street comes a tall man with a large gait, walking quickly. Over his shoulders he drapes a large, colorful blanket flowing around him. He bounces with his quick gait.

The man has several days of whiskers decorating his face, and he looks like he has spent a bitterly cold night over a warm heat grate along the underground Metro line. His long, tangled hair and dirty clothes mark him as a saint of winter, one of the few souls who had left the crowded shelter. The leftover smile across his active face shines in the bitter cold. This morning a strange figure blew down a winter street on the fifth day of January 2001.

Sometimes I shut my eyes and I see, not darkness, but unknown men and women standing before a house, captured in a stiff photo of long ago. I recognize none of the faces staring with fresh smiles. Why can't I remember who they are? Did I ever know them with any intimacy, or are they shards of memory, damaged and abandoned to die?

Torn papers and rusty leaves dance down the sidewalks as I walk through a winter morning, whipped by cold, unsteady breezes.

My cat Sabina possesses electric eyes that stare out of the dark bedroom, an aberration from another planet with a steady green/yellow gaze. This little cat with the thick misty coat of gray is my guardian since I fell under the control of Alzheimer's. It was at that time she came in the dark night bedroom and sat at the end of my bed, a sentinel to protect me from other deadly marauders hovering over me at night when I was helplessly asleep.

She watches the door with intensity as a thin strip of light insinuates its way into the bedroom like a silent thief.

Sabina took up guarding me soon after she recovered from near death at the hands of a clumsy veterinarian. Joyce and I nursed her back to the living from trembling fear. Those were frightening days when Sabina was on the edge of death. When she recovered, she took to sleeping on my bed at night. I like to think she is paying me back now that I suffer under the death knell, waiting for Alzheimer's to slip through the thin, dark night and steal me away to the place of hot ashes and emptiness.

There are days during which I am happier than ever, full of real joy, despite the slow death unwinding itself inside my brain.

At night, in the silent darkness, I lie down on the sofa and place myself carefully to see airplanes coasting in the darkness as they settle like fairies into National Airport several miles away.

To me, from where I watch, the planes are more than lights twinkling like fast-moving stars lumbering toward a landing. From where I lie in watch, I lose sight of them quickly. There is often a steady march of these silent wingless lights following their downward trajectories, but I am never able to view a landing from my sofa.

My nights are empty, as are my days, waiting here for the end to come. Apart from the moments of movement in the night air, there is only the deadly flickering of the television to comfort me.

In the depth of winter I watch snow fill the air thickly. The day is gray and forbidding, but the snow brings a festive feel and my heart beats rapidly with happiness. There is nothing I like better than a walk in a snow shower, and time to forget.

*   *   *

Our house on Ivy Street has the look of a wild forgotten place. Weeds wander where there were once graveled walks. In the outdoor garden beds, the once lovely, well-tended plants are besieged by uninvited growth. The place does not sparkle as it did in earlier years. It is now full of the secrets of dying. The empty landscape is the victim of time and the people who brought change.

In earlier times, the house was bright and neat. In the back-yard, a manicured garden produced red tomatoes, green and gold peppers, sassy sorrel, sweet lavenders, aromatic thymes and pungent rosemary. The cherry tree that was only a sapling when it first occupied this land is now a rough, dark, dead obelisk, slowly rotting on the spot from which it sprang many years ago.

A large greenhouse covers most of the backyard. Today it slumbers in the sun, shaded by trembling bamboo, now taller than a two-story house. A former next-door neighbor planted this out-of-context green nuisance years ago in an unsuccessful effort to thwart my dream of becoming an urban farmer. He thought the bamboo's heavy shadow created so much shade my plants would fail.

He watched as Francesco and I spent a summer digging a deep ditch the length of the property, three feet deep in heavy clay soil. We installed a heavy weed barrier on our side of his fence to stop the fickle penetration of his bamboo into our lives.

Inside the greenhouse, a sense of loss highlighted with tat-tooed memories stretches to meet the midday sun. Dead and dying plants lie in the deep shadows under the heavy wire benches. The place is in decline, as is its owner, and fresh weeds cover the pebbled earth.

This large greenhouse is no longer used. It is emptied of questions and laughter that filled it when the plant business was bustling. Now I am sick, weary and full of uncertainty. I am possessed by stuttering dreams and lackadaisical memory.

Yesterday has no meaning anymore. Events of today flee

from memory before day concludes. My brain is full of forgotten memories. The few remaining memories are scars of long ago. I live in the moment now. I remember I had a past but it is vacant now in a time of sorrow.

Alzheimer's is a deadly hole in my life, a deep cistern into which I tripped unknowingly. I am spinning out of control as I fall through the wet darkness. When I hit the water, I begin to sink to the bottom where the abyss greets me. I sit still, waiting for the moment I can no longer breathe.

Time is coming apart in my rough hands. An end begins to circle me. Let me hug this woman, my wife who has stood beside me for so many trembling years. I salute my son with a hug this one last time before darkness comes. Goodbye, Joyce. So long, Francesco.

On dark streets it is difficult to see the faces of those walking past, especially on cold blustery days with yanked-down hats and toasty mufflers. On clear summer days the fear of death is sometimes palpable, running down sunburned cheeks.

The fear of death is everywhere, but unseen. It is under the coats of those stiff-faced, mysterious people who populate the sidewalks as they leave work. A glut of fear inhabits the soft places where no one wants to look. A man like me is appointed to excavate these sly places as he lopes toward death.

Death is a challenge for beings who can feel their own demise squirming in a deteriorating body. After you feel death crawling inside, and watch it scamper over hallucinating dark night walls, there is no reason to have fear. In the end, death does not matter; it lightens the earth's load, and enriches those who follow.

White gulls sweep from the sky. In a moment they soar to new heights on warm, familiar currents, as cars speed beneath them.

A single man proceeds along the sidewalk as he has every morning for several dozen years. His gait is crisp and it lends a sense of purpose to what has been a solitary lark for years.

As the walker comes to a turning point, he adjusts his cap low on his head, preparing to look into the bright rising sun.

Balloons dance over electric lights high above the street.

About the Author

THOMAS DEBAGGIO has worked as both a professional herb grower and a newspaper journalist. He is the author of *Losing My Mind* and of *Growing Herbs from Seed, Cutting & Root, Basil: An Herb Lover's Guide* (with Susan Belsinger), and *The Big Book of Herbs* (with Arthur O. Tucker). He lives with his wife in Arlington, Virginia.